Textbook of Advanced Dermatology: Pearls for Academia and Skin Clinics

(Part 1)

Edited by

Mohammad Reza Namazi
*Shiraz University of Medical Sciences and
Dr. Namazi Skin and Hair Clinic, Shiraz, Iran*

Textbook of Advanced Dermatology: Pearls for Academia and Skin Clinics (Part 1)

Editor: Mohammad Reza Namazi

ISBN (Online): 978-981-5223-52-1

ISBN (Print): 978-981-5223-53-8

ISBN (Paperback): 978-981-5223-54-5

First published in 2024.

need for a court order if at any point you breach any terms of this License Agreement. In no event will any delay or failure by Bentham Science Publishers in enforcing your compliance with this License Agreement constitute a waiver of any of its rights.

3. You acknowledge that you have read this License Agreement, and agree to be bound by its terms and conditions. To the extent that any other terms and conditions presented on any website of Bentham Science Publishers conflict with, or are inconsistent with, the terms and conditions set out in this License Agreement, you acknowledge that the terms and conditions set out in this License Agreement shall prevail.

Bentham Science Publishers Pte. Ltd.
80 Robinson Road #02-00
Singapore 068898
Singapore
Email: subscriptions@benthamscience.net

BENTHAM SCIENCE

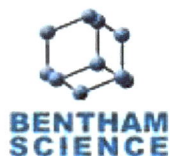

CONTENTS

PREFACE i

LIST OF CONTRIBUTORS iii

DEDICATION iv

CHAPTER 1 INTRODUCTION 1
Mohammad Reza Namazi

PART 1 TEACHING PEARLS

**CHAPTER 2 INTERESTING WAYS TO ENCOURAGE TRAINEES FOR PROPER
HISTORY TAKING AND PHYSICAL EXAMINATION** 3
Mohammad Reza Namazi
REFERENCES 6

**CHAPTER 3 TWO BIG TEACHING MISTAKES THAT YOUNG ASSISTANT
PROFESSORS/CONSULTANTS MAY MAKE** 7
Mohammad Reza Namazi
REFERENCES 9

CHAPTER 4 UNKNOWN SLIDES: VERY USEFUL TEACHING MATERIALS 10
Mohammad Reza Namazi

PART 2 MEDICAL PEARLS

CHAPTER 5 PRACTICAL WAYS TO IMPROVE PATIENT ADHERENCE 11
Megan Mukenge, Christina Kontzias and *Steven R. Feldman*
REFERENCES 13

CHAPTER 6 MOISTURIZER PEARLS 14
Mohammad Reza Namazi
REFERENCES 16

**CHAPTER 7 HOW TO MAKE AN OILY CALAMINE COMPOUND WHICH DOES NOT
DRY THE SKIN?** 18
Mohammad Reza Namazi
REFERENCES 18

CHAPTER 8 HOW TO MAKE STRONG TOPICAL ANTI-ITCH COMPOUNDS? 19
Mohammad Reza Namazi
REFERENCES 20

CHAPTER 9 TOPICAL STEROIDS AND STEROID VEHICLES: SOME PEARLS 21
Mohammad Reza Namazi
REFERENCES 22

CHAPTER 10 STEROIDS: SOME PEARLS 23
Mohammad Reza Namazi
REFERENCES 24

CHAPTER 11 STEROID COMPARISON TABLE 25
Mohammad Reza Namazi
REFERENCES 26

CHAPTER 12 PULSE STEROID THERAPY 27
Mohammad Reza Namazi
REFERENCES 28

CHAPTER 13 INTRADERMAL TRIAMCINOLONE INJECTION 29

Mohammad Reza Namazi

REFERENCE 30

CHAPTER 14 INCREASING THE EFFICACY OF INTRAVENOUS N-ACETYLCYSTEINE ... 31

Mohammad Reza Namazi

REFERENCES 31

CHAPTER 15 POSTHERPETIC NEURALGIA: PEARLS 32

Mohammad Reza Namazi

REFERENCES 33

**CHAPTER 16 AN IMPORTANT POINT IN INTRAVENOUS ACYCLOVIR
ADMINISTRATION** 34

Mohammad Reza Namazi

REFERENCES 34

CHAPTER 17 GENITAL WARTS: PEARLS 35

Mohammad Reza Namazi

REFERENCES 39

**CHAPTER 18 UPTON'S PASTE: AN EXTREMELY POTENT COMPOUND FOR
RESISTANT WARTS, CALLOUSES AND CORNS** 41

Mohammad Reza Namazi

REFERENCE 42

**CHAPTER 19 GOOD KERATOLYTICS FOR NON-IRRITATED THICK SKIN, E.G.,
LICHEN SIMPLEX CHRONICUS AND KERATOSIS PILARIS** 43

Mohammad Reza Namazi

REFERENCE 44

CHAPTER 20 ANTI-HISTAMINES PEARLS 45

Mohammad Reza Namazi

REFERENCES 46

CHAPTER 21 ACNE MANAGEMENT: PEARLS 47

Mohammad Reza Namazi

REFERENCES 48

**CHAPTER 22 WHICH TOPICALS ARE APPROPRIATE FOR ACNE PATIENTS WITH
DRY SKIN?** 49

Mohammad Reza Namazi

REFERENCE 50

CHAPTER 23 MELASMA PEARLS 51

Mohammad Reza Namazi

REFERENCES 53

CHAPTER 24 HOW TO MAKE A STRONG ANTI-ACNE AND ANTI-PIGMENT AGENT? ... 54

Mohammad Reza Namazi

REFERENCES 54

**CHAPTER 25 HOW TO TREAT PERI-ORBITAL HYPERMELANOSIS AND MELASMA IN
SENSITIVE SKIN?** 55

Mohammad Reza Namazi

REFERENCES 55

CHAPTER 26 DOXYCYCLINE OR AZITHROMYCIN FOR PERIFOLLICULAR ELASTOLYSIS? 56
   Mohammad Reza Namazi
   REFERENCES 56

CHAPTER 27 EXCESSIVE SKIN OILINESS: TIPS 57
   Mohammad Reza Namazi
   REFERENCES 58

CHAPTER 28 ENLARGED PORES 59
   Mohammad Reza Namazi
   REFERENCE 59

CHAPTER 29 FACIAL ERYTHEMA 60
   Mohammad Reza Namazi
   REFERENCES 61

CHAPTER 30 WHAT IS AN EXCELLENT ANTI-REDNESS EMOLLIENT FOR ICHTHYOSIFORM ERYTHRODERMA? 62
   Mohammad Reza Namazi
   REFERENCES 63

CHAPTER 31 PEMPHIGUS PEARLS 64
   Mohammad Reza Namazi
   REFERENCES 66

CHAPTER 32 PATHERGY TESTING FOR DIAGNOSING BEHCET'S DISEASE 68
   Mohammad Reza Namazi1,* 68
   REFERENCE 69

CHAPTER 33 MILD-TO-MODERATE PSORIASIS TIPS 70
   Alyssa Curcio, Christina Kontzias and *Steven R. Feldman*
   REFERENCES 72

CHAPTER 34 SEVERE PSORIASIS: PEARLS 74
   Mohammad Reza Namazi
   REFERENCES 76

CHAPTER 35 SEBORRHEIC DERMATITIS TIPS 77
   Mohammad Reza Namazi
   REFERENCES 78

CHAPTER 36 WOUND VAC AND HYPERBARIC OXYGEN FOR WOUND HEALING 79
   Mohammad Reza Namazi
   REFERENCES 80

CHAPTER 37 SOME TIPS ON HEAD LICE MANAGEMENT 81
   Mohammad Reza Namazi
   REFERENCES 82

CHAPTER 38 CUTANEOUS LEISHMANIASIS PEARLS 83
   Mohammad Reza Namazi
   REFERENCES 85

CHAPTER 39 ALOPECIA AREATA: SOME TIPS 87
   Mohammad Reza Namazi
   REFERENCES 88

CHAPTER 40 THE BENEFITS OF POTASSIUM PERMANGANATE 89
Mohammad Reza Namazi
REFERENCES 90

CHAPTER 41 STRENGTHENING THE IMMUNE RESPONSE 91
Mohammad Reza Namazi
REFERENCES 92

CHAPTER 42 MACULAR AMYLOIDOSIS PEARLS 93
Mohammad Reza Namazi
REFERENCES 93

CHAPTER 43 MYCOSIS FUNGOIDES PEARLS 94
Mohammad Reza Namazi
REFERENCES 95

**CHAPTER 44 THE PRO-OXIDANT ACTIVITY OF ANTI-OXIDANTS AND ITS
PRACTICAL IMPLICATIONS** 96
Mohammad Reza Namazi
REFERENCES 97

CHAPTER 45 HOW TO PREVENT THE GROWTH OF NEUROFIBROMAS? 98
Mohammad Reza Namazi
REFERENCES 98

CHAPTER 46 HOW TO EXPEDITE DEPIGMENTATION THERAPY IN VITILIGO? 99
Mohammad Reza Namazi
REFERENCES 99

CHAPTER 47 THE PROBLEM IN DIAGNOSING EARLY VITILIGO 100
Mohammad Reza Namazi
REFERENCES 100

CHAPTER 48 VITILIGO PEARLS 101
Mohammad Reza Namazi
REFERENCES 103

CHAPTER 49 TIPS TO PREVENT HAIR DAMAGE 104
Mohammad Reza Namazi
REFERENCES 105

CHAPTER 50 ANDROGENETIC HAIR LOSS: SOME IMPORTANT MANAGEMENT TIPS 106
Mohammad Reza Namazi
REFERENCES 109

CHAPTER 51 TELOGEN EFFLUVIUM: TIPS 111
Mohammad Reza Namazi
REFERENCES 112

**CHAPTER 52 FRONTAL FIBROSING ALOPECIA/LICHEN PLANOPILARIS: SOME
PEARLS** 113
Mohammad Reza Namazi
REFERENCES 115

CHAPTER 53 METHOTREXATE PEARLS 116
Mohammad Reza Namazi
REFERENCES 117

CHAPTER 54 INTRAVENOUS IMMUNOGLOBULIN PEARLS 118
Mohammad Reza Namazi
REFERENCES 119

CHAPTER 55 A SIMPLE, LIMITED PATCH TESTING 121
Mohammad Reza Namazi
REFERENCES 122

CHAPTER 56 WET WRAP 123
Mohammad Reza Namazi
REFERENCES 124

CHAPTER 57 MANAGEMENT OF VARICOSE VEINS 125
Mohammad Reza Namazi
REFERENCES 127

CHAPTER 58 IMPROVING SCAR FORMATION: PEARLS 129
Mohammad Reza Namazi
REFERENCES 130

CHAPTER 59 MISCELLANEOUS MEDICAL PEARLS 133
Mohammad Reza Namazi
REFERENCES 138

PART 3 PUBLICATION PEARLS

CHAPTER 60 PUBLICATION PEARLS 139
Mohammad Reza Namazi

SUBJECT INDEX 145

PREFACE

"My intentions are to spread knowledge; I consider this the most important happiness."

Biruni, a Persian encyclopedic scientist

"Our writings will remain, while we will go. Nothing will remain in the world from us except our writings."

Ferdowsi, a Persian giant poet

"Do not coil on the treasure of science like a snake and deprive science-seekers from acquiring it."

Ali-ibn-Abitaleb, an Arab leader

During my 20-year dermatology practice, including my residency period, I have frequently encountered important clinical challenges that could not be solved by referring to major dermatology textbooks, making me search dermatology papers and the less well-known books to solve these problems. Also, during the past two decades, I have been practicing both medical and procedural dermatology as well as conducting research and writing papers; therefore, I have gained a lot of experience which is not mentioned anywhere. Not to mention my experience in teaching as a university academic staff and in business as a founder and director of my private dermatology clinic.

I thought it would be a big pity not to share the interesting practical points I learned and also my laboriously achieved experience with my colleagues and future dermatologists, believing that any person should write at least one book during his lifetime to share his unique experience with his/her fellow human beings. Actually, this was the motivation to start writing this book. Later on, I became interested in encouraging the collaboration of other colleagues, some being the world leaders in their specific fields, to strengthen this book. I would like to extend my deep gratitude to these dear colleagues who have greatly honored me with their marvelous contributions.

The present book is composed of 5 sections: Teaching Pearls, Medical Pearls, Procedural Pearls, Publication Pearls, and Business Pearls, therefore, encompassing the broad realm of dermatology and filling the large gap in the major dermatology textbooks. Importantly, this book does not aim to provide detailed information on each topic, rather it aims to provide interesting tips which cannot be found or can hardly be found elsewhere. **Therefore, as an advanced dermatology textbook, much important essential information that can easily be obtained from other publications is not included in this book**.

I would like to thank all my dear colleagues who have kindly referred surgical patients to me, especially Drs. Ali Mohammad Namiyan, Amir Kalafi, Mahsa Naseri, Masoud Koraee, Ahmad Moradi, Arash Abtahiyan, Yasaam Khosravi, Khalil Hamedpour and other colleagues whom I may not remember.

I would also like to thank my assistants, Mr. Mohammad Khanchefalak and Ms. Bahar Bayat, for their help in taking photos and Prof. Nasrin Shokrpour for editing some parts of this book.

This preface cannot be concluded without sincerely thanking Bentham's publishing staff, especially Miss Humaira Hashmi, Ms. Simra Nasir and Ms. Ambreen Irshad, for their help in making the dream of this book a reality.

"This well-arranged composition will remain for years, When every atom of our dust is dispersed.

The intention of this design was that it should survive

Because I perceive no stability in my existence…"

This poem is from Saadi Shirazi, a great Persian poet (translated by Edward Rehatsek into English).

Mohammad Reza Namazi
Shiraz University of Medical Sciences and
Dr. Namazi Skin and Hair Clinic, Shiraz, Iran

List of Contributors

Mohammad Reza Namazi Shiraz University of Medical Sciences and Dr. Namazi Skin and Hair Clinic, Shiraz, Iran

Megan Mukenge Center for Dermatology Research, Department of Dermatology, Wake Forest School of Medicine, Winston-Salem, North Carolina, USA

Christina Kontzias Center for Dermatology Research, Department of Dermatology, Wake Forest School of Medicine, Winston-Salem, North Carolina, USA

Steven R. Feldman Department of Social Sciences & Health Policy, Wake Forest School of Medicine, Winston-Salem, North Carolina, USA

Alyssa Curcio Center for Dermatology Research, Department of Dermatology, Wake Forest School of Medicine, Winston-Salem, North Carolina, USA

DEDICATION

To Drs. Uranus Dasmeh, Aliakbar Mohammadi, Vahid Dastgerdi, plastic surgeons in Shiraz, Iran and Dr. Mohsen Alirezai, dermatologist and plastic surgeon in Montpellier, France, for responding to my consultations and queries; Dr. Manouchr Sodaifi, founder of the Dermatology Department of Shiraz University of Medical Sciences, for his amazing interest in teaching; and Dr. Behrooz Kasraee for his help.

To my dear wife Masoumeh, who got headaches on weekends from the constant sound of typing this book from dawn to dusk, and our beloved flowers Sahand and Anahid.

To the memory of Prof. Karim Vessal, the Father of Iran's Modern Medical Editing:

"Near, far, wherever you are, I believe that the heart does go on...

You are safe in our hearts, and our hearts will go on and on..."

CHAPTER 1

Introduction

Mohammad Reza Namazi[1,*]

[1] *Shiraz University of Medical Sciences and Dr. Namazi Skin and Hair Clinic, Shiraz, Iran*

Dermatology seems to be originated from internal medicine. The older generation of dermatologists was mainly involved in treating skin diseases. However, this field has progressed tremendously during the past decades, advancing its procedural part to include many surgical operations that were traditionally believed to lie within the realm of plastic surgery.

On the other hand, the progress in laser technology has dramatically advanced the borders of dermatology. A few decades ago, thinking about the use of laser in dermatology was just like science fiction.

Since dermatology is a lucrative field, especially its aesthetic and procedural parts, other physicians, such as general practitioners and even some specialists, have been lured to undertake many non-invasive or minimally invasive procedures that dermatologists believe to belong to their field. This has led to a fierce competition, and the winner of this competition, being cut-throat in some countries, is perhaps the person who not only masters the aforementioned procedures but also knows the business acumen. Unfortunately, business issues, while important, are not taught in the residency period, and there are many expert dermatologists who end up working in clinics belonging to businessmen because they do not know the business acumen.

In this book, besides the purely academic parts of dermatology, *i.e.*, teaching and research, other sections of this wide discipline, *i.e.*, medical, aesthetic and procedural parts, are also covered, and a separate section is also devoted to the business tips.

In the medical section, many compounding formulations of topical compounds are provided. These are mainly based on the author's experience in the prescription of topical compounds. The prescription of topical compounds is done for several reasons. Firstly, the available commercial products may not contain all the ingre-

* **Corresponding author Mohammad Reza Namazi:** Shiraz University of Medical Sciences and Dr. Namazi Skin and Hair Clinic, Shiraz, Iran; E-mail: rezanamazi12@yahoo.com

dients effective against different pathophysiologic aspects of a condition. This may be due to the novelty of a compounding formula or the fact that compounding on an industrial scale is so difficult compared to that on a small scale performed in a local pharmacy. Secondly, the commercial products may not have the required ingredients at the concentrations a dermatologist prefers. Thirdly, to have an adequate shelf-life, preservatives are added to commercial products, which can negatively affect the skin, especially sensitive skin. Finally, there are some patients who would rather use a prescription compound than a commercial product because they are fed up or disappointed with the latter, or they think prescription compounds are stronger. Therefore, knowing compounding formulations is a must for every competent dermatologist and is usually a distinguishing feature from a general practitioner.

I hope the readers find the tips provided in this textbook useful.

Teaching Pearls

CHAPTER 2

Interesting Ways to Encourage Trainees for Proper History Taking and Physical Examination

Mohammad Reza Namazi[1,*]

[1] *Shiraz University of Medical Sciences and Dr. Namazi Skin and Hair Clinic, Shiraz, Iran*

Developing the trainees' observation skills and encouraging them to spend adequate time on meticulous history taking and physical examination are not done easily. Two interesting tips to achieve these goals are presented:

-Tell the story of Al-Bakri, the great traveler of mind:

Al-Bakri was born in Spain (1040-1094 CE). He received travelers and merchants in his home and interpreted their stories into his "Book of Highways and Kingdoms". He made accurate references to the geography, culture, religion and trade of Europe, North Africa and the Arabian Peninsula, all this without ever traveling to these distant lands himself! [1] The crater Al-Bakri on the Moon is named after him [2]. Al-Bakri is perhaps the greatest history taker in human history.

A giant semblance of Al-Bakri was displayed at Expo 2020 in Dubai (Fig. **1**).

- The Sherlock Holmes series and stories can serve as excellent astuteness inspirers for medical trainees. Sherlock Holmes is a fictional supersleuth who greatly stresses on keen observation, meticulous inspection and heeding details and apparent trifles, which are especially related to dermatological practice. It has been appropriately said that a dermatologist should be a proficient detective possessing the powers of observation and deduction when facing contact dermatitis [3]. In "The Adventure of the Blanched Soldier", Holmes states that he has the habit of sitting with his back to the window while seating his clients in the opposite chair where the light falls fully upon them. Dermatological practice in the gaslight era was exactly the same. Additionally, the dermatologist must have enough exposure of the skin, not trusting the patient's assurance that lesions are or are not present in an area or that they are similar or dissimilar to the ones that

---

[*] **Corresponding author Mohammad Reza Namazi:** Shiraz University of Medical Sciences and Dr. Namazi Skin and Hair Clinic, Shiraz, Iran; E-mail: rezanamazi12@yahoo.com

have been shown. "There is nothing like first-hand evidence," says Holmes in "A Study in Scarlet". He disapproves of theorising on inadequate data in "The Valley of Fear". The dermatologic examination needs the highest alertness. In "The Hound of the Baskervilles", Holmes states that "The world is full of obvious things that nobody by any chance ever observes" [4].

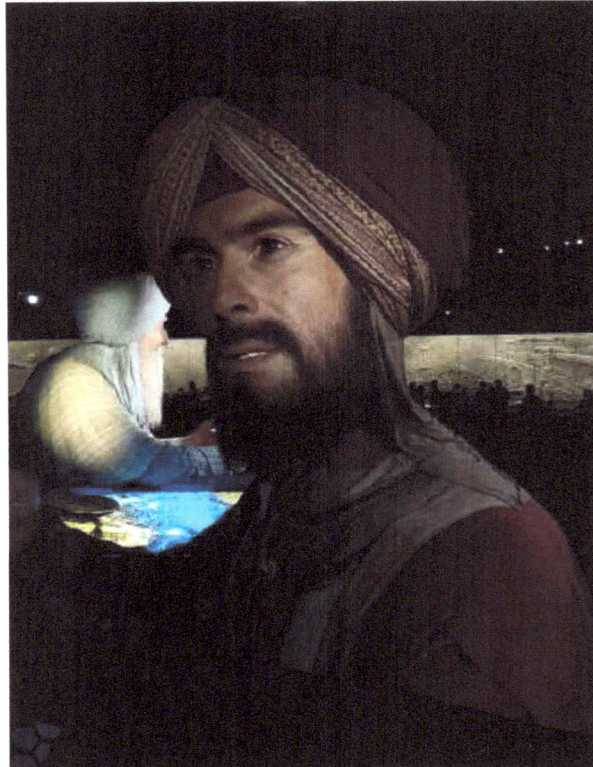

Fig. (l). Al-Bakri's giant semblance in Expo 2020, Dubai.

William Bennett Bean, a professor of medicine and the Chair of Internal Medicine at the College of Medicine, University of Iowa, wrote that novices in medicine should master Sherlock Holmes [5]. Ira Martin Grais, a cardiologist at Northwestern University Feinberg School of Medicine in Chicago, mentioned that during the 5 decades of teaching in medical schools, he had made the reading of certain Sherlock Holmes stories mandatory for the trainees [6].

In 1885, Dr. Arthur Conan Doyle, a young physician, created Sherlock Holmes, modeled upon a Scottish lecturer and surgeon at the University of Edinburgh, Dr. Joseph Bell, who stressed the importance of careful observation in making a diagnosis. To demonstrate this, he often chose a stranger and deduced his job and recent activities by observing him. He would surprise his students with his intuitive powers and sharp observation skills and stressed the significance of developing students' observant faculties [3].

Sherlock Holmes stories are very influential and interesting, especially for young people. A paper published in the *Journal of Dermatology and Surgical Oncology* in 1979 [4], *i.e.*, 93 years after the creation of Sherlock Holmes, mentioned that "Hundreds of letters are still addressed to him [at 221B Baker Street, London] each year, asking for help or advice!"

The Sherlock Holmes Society of London, founded in 1951, publishes Sherlock Holmes Journal twice a year and has erected a big statue of him in London (Fig. **2**). The Sherlock Holmes Museum (Fig. **3**) was opened in 1990 in Baker Street and features some items from several different adaptations of Sherlock Holmes. A PubMed search for papers having "Sherlock Holmes" in their titles/abstracts revealed 182 results at the time of writing this text (10 March 2023), including some papers published in 2023.

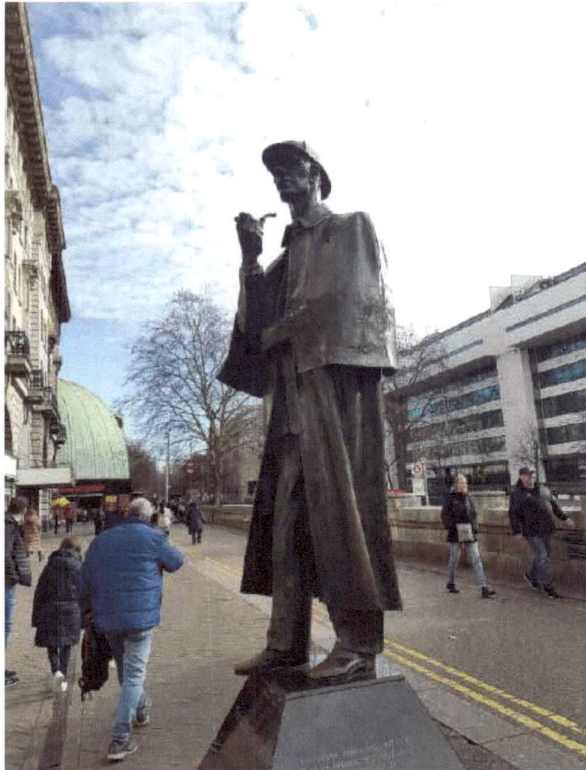

Fig. (2). Sherlock Holmes' Colossus in London.

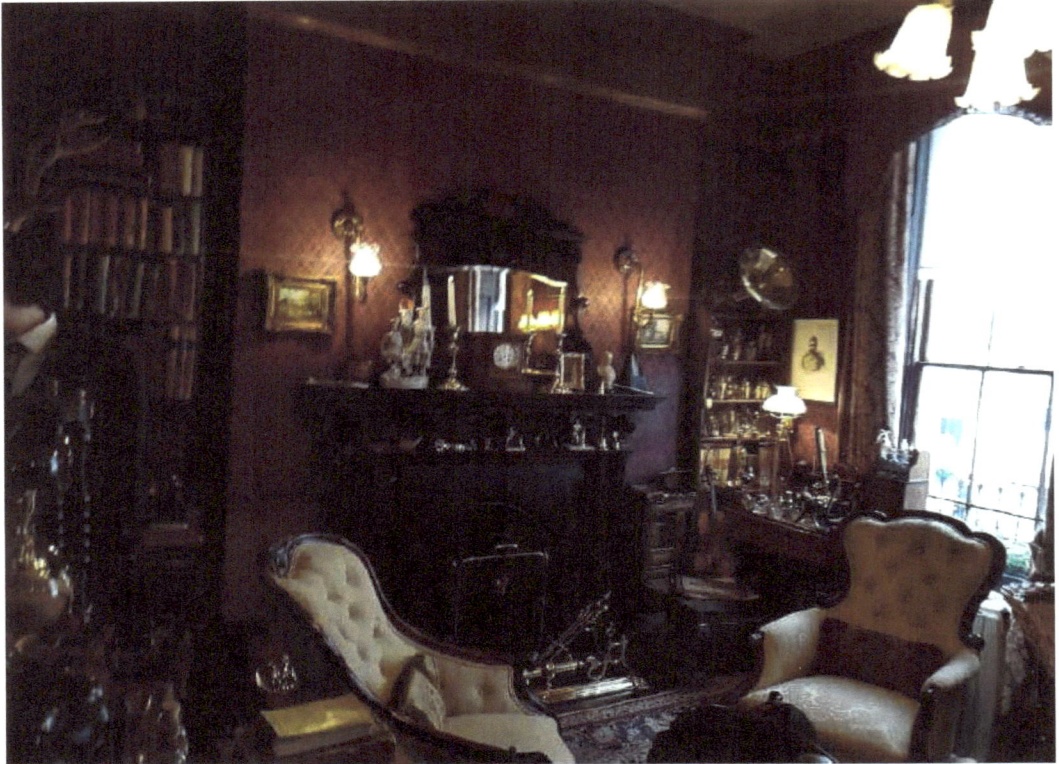

Fig. (3). Sherlock Holm's Museum in London. Holmes asserted his habit of sitting with his back to the window while seating his clients in the opposite chair with the light falling fully on them.

REFERENCES

[1]   Lévi-Provençal E, Abū U. Encyclopaedia of Islam. 2nd. Leiden: Brill 1960; 1: pp. 155-7.

[2]   Gazetteer of Planetary Nomenclature. https://planetarynames.wr.usgs.gov/Feature/145. Accessed: 12/9/2022.

[3]   Klauder JV. Sherlock Holmes as a dermatologist, with remarks on the life of Dr. Joseph Bell and the Sherlockian method of teaching. AMA Arch Derm Syphilol. 1953 Oct; 68(4): 363-77.

[4]   Dirckx JH. Medicine and literature: Sherlock Holmes and the art of dermatologic diagnosis. J Dermatol Surg Oncol. 1979 Mar; 5(3): 191-6 4.

[5]   Bean WB. The private life of Sherlock Holmes by Vincent Starrett [book review]. Arch Intern Med 1962; 110(6): 926-7.

[6]   Grais IM. False scents, false sense, and false cents: why physicians should read Sherlock Holmes. Tex Heart Inst J. 2012; 39(3): 319-21.

CHAPTER 3

Two Big Teaching Mistakes that Young Assistant Professors/Consultants May Make

Mohammad Reza Namazi[1,*]

[1] *Shiraz University of Medical Sciences and Dr. Namazi Skin and Hair Clinic, Shiraz, Iran*

Herein, I tell the story of the two mistakes I made while I was a young Assistant Professor in order to help my colleagues promote their teaching methods.

At the start of my career at the university as an Assistant Professor, I thought that I should encourage the trainees to study more by asking them tough questions that could not be answered by them and then reprimanding them for not knowing the answer. I thought the pain inflicted by my criticism would stimulate them to study more and gain more knowledge. Though this may be true, it was not a good approach as it was distressing for them, making them not like me and attend my classes and clinics with alacrity. Moreover, in many situations, I asked them unimportant, difficult questions, *e.g.*, the percentages mentioned in textbooks of various manifestations of a disease, to achieve my goal, which was a waste of time, of course.

While I was a fellow in the prestigious dermatology department of Wake-Forest University, USA, I learned an interesting, completely opposite approach from Prof. Omar Sangueza, a famous dermatopathologist and the Editor-in-Chief of the American Journal of Dermatopathology. Unlike me, he asked the residents only important questions and gave energizing, positive feedback to those who answered correctly by saying: "You are completely right [with a high intonation]. The diagnosis is…"

B.F. Skinner, one of the most influential psychologists of the 20th century, has shown that an animal who is rewarded for a wanted behavior learns that behavior more rapidly than an animal who is punished for an unwanted behavior. This can be applicable to teaching humans. Criticisms cause resentment and even hatred. Instead, be positive and encourage people [1].

* **Corresponding author Mohammad Reza Namazi:** Shiraz University of Medical Sciences and Dr. Namazi Skin and Hair Clinic, Shiraz, Iran; E-mail: rezanamazi12@yahoo.com

The second mistake I used to make was to dominate my teaching at dermatology rounds with basic science materials, including very complex subjects, because I loved basic sciences. I asked the residents and even the medical students difficult questions regarding the pathophysiology of diseases and cellular and molecular medicine. Most of them disliked these topics; they were mainly interested in clinical and practical subjects. With time, I learned to dominate my discussions with practical materials, mentioning only very important basic science subjects having practical implications. The following sentences from the book "How to Win Friends and Influence People", the seventh most influential book in American history written by Dale Carnegie (Fig. **1**), deserve careful consideration:

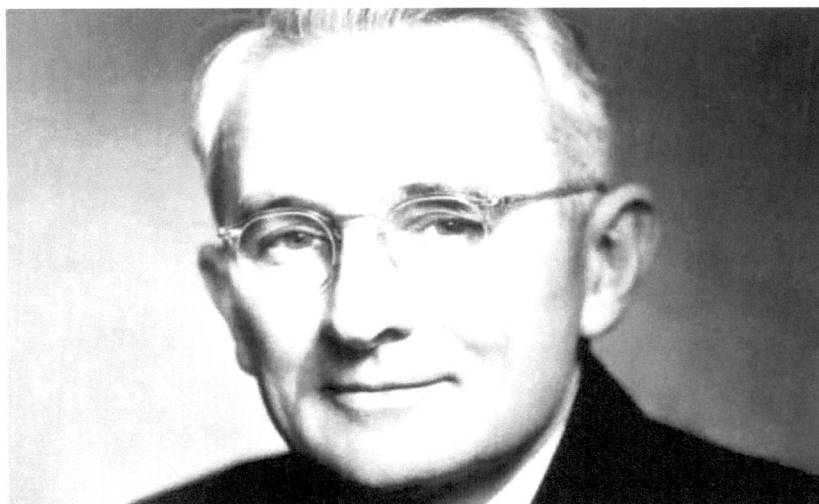

Fig. (1). Dale Carnegie, the American writer whose book *"How to Win Friends and Influence People"* had sold five million copies in 31 languages by the time of his death.

"I often went fishing up in Maine during the summer. Personally, I am very fond of strawberries and cream, but I have found that, for some strange reason, fish prefer worms. So when I went fishing, I didn't think about what I wanted. I thought about what they wanted. I didn't bait the hook with strawberries and cream. Rather, I dangled a worm or a grasshopper in front of the fish and said: "Wouldn't you like to have that?" Why not use the same common sense when fishing for people?

Why talk about what we want? That is childish. Absurd. Of course, you are interested in what you want. You are eternally interested in it. But no one else is. The rest of us are just like you: we are interested in what we want." [2].

REFERENCES

[1]   Carnegie D. How to Win Friends and Influence People?. 9th ed. Tehran: Peyman Publisher 2009; p. 24.

[2]   Carnegie D. How to Win Friends and Influence People?. Revised edition. New York: Simon and Schuster 1981; p. 46.

CHAPTER 4

Unknown Slides: Very Useful Teaching Materials

Mohammad Reza Namazi[1,*]

[1] *Shiraz University of Medical Sciences and Dr. Namazi Skin and Hair Clinic, Shiraz, Iran*

Knowing impactful teaching methods can dramatically enhance your teaching capability.

A remarkable teaching method I noticed at the Department of Dermatology at Wake Forest University, USA, was the use of unknown slides. Several slides with no diagnoses were placed in a room near a microscope at the beginning of each week. Residents had the chance to see them and guess the diagnoses prior to discussing the correct diagnoses by the pathologists at the end of the week.

[*] **Corresponding author Mohammad Reza Namazi:** Shiraz University of Medical Sciences and Dr. Namazi Skin and Hair Clinic, Shiraz, Iran; E-mail: rezanamazi12@yahoo.com

Medical Pearls

CHAPTER 5

Practical Ways to Improve Patient Adherence

Megan Mukenge[1], **Christina Kontzias**[1] and **Steven R. Feldman**[1,*]

[1] *Center for Dermatology Research, Department of Dermatology, Wake Forest School of Medicine, Winston-Salem, North Carolina, USA*

Patient adherence involves collaboration between the patients and their providers. Poor adherence can negatively impact clinical outcomes and increase frustration among patients. Provided are pearls for promoting patient adherence:

-Assessing adherence can be challenging. It may be tempting to ask if patients are taking their medications as prescribed. Often, patients answer based on what they think we want to hear. Consider opting for an indirect line of questioning that can lead to a more truthful response. For example, ask patients, "How and/or when do you take your medication?" or "How many days a week you are not able to take your medication?" Also, you can suggest that patients bring their medications to each office visit. However, this could yield misleading information as patients may discard their medication before the visit.

-Patients are more diligent in following their treatment plans in the days leading up to their appointment and shortly after the office visit [1]. This trend can be explained by white coat compliance. Therefore, implementing strategies that increase the frequency of follow-up visits could be beneficial in improving adherence. Minimizing follow-up time should be considered for initial visits, especially when prescribing a new treatment regimen. If this is not practical, consider virtual assessments. When appropriate, consider progress photo submissions. When patients require less frequent monitoring, consider extending the follow-up time.

-Engage the patients as much as possible when creating a treatment plan. When patients feel included in decision-making, they tend to foster a greater sense of ownership in their health. This can strengthen the physician-patient relationship

---

* **Corresponding author Steven R. Feldman:** Department of Social Sciences & Health Policy, Wake Forest School of Medicine, Winston- Salem, North Carolina, USA; E-mail: sfeldman@wakehealth.edu

Mohammad Reza Namazi (Ed.)

by building upon the trust and accountability fundamental in promoting adherence.

-Providing samples of topical therapies is a helpful strategy when initiating treatment. This allows the patient to experience the differences between vehicles (*i.e.*, cream versus ointment) and can build rapport with the provider because it involves them in the decision-making process.

-A simplified treatment plan is advantageous in improving adherence. Complex treatment plans can be overwhelming for patients, particularly when they have to remember when and how to use multiple medications throughout the day. Opting for a less complicated plan that focuses on consistently using one or two medications could be more favorable. The use of combination drugs may also be helpful. Providers should also be mindful of medication costs, as expensive medications can deter patients from filling their prescriptions. Inform patients to follow up if the drug is costly so you can explore other options with them. Also, inquiring about patients' daily schedules and priorities can be helpful when designing a treatment plan.

-Strive to give patients written instructions on how to use their medication(s). Encourage patients to keep this information on their dresser, bathroom mirror, refrigerator door, or somewhere visible to remind them to use their medications. You can also upload a copy of the written instructions to the patient's electronic chart and/or have the patient take a photo of the instructions so that the information is still accessible if they lose the original copy.

-Fear plays an instrumental role in dictating behavior. Recognizing and validating patients' emotional states can assist in reframing their perspective on potential adverse events associated with all medications. Properly educating patients on potential side effects and providing patients with appropriate action plans if these effects arise can improve adherence and safety. For patients who fear they will be the sole person who develops a rare side effect, explaining that the majority of people taking the medication do not develop the side effect could be enough to change their mind. We can also use side effects in our favor to indicate the medicine is working appropriately, which can serve as a motivational tool for patients to continue treatment. For example, we can counsel a patient starting on topical retinoid for acne to push through the dryness phase, as this is a sign the medication is working.

-For patients starting on injectable biologics, the anchoring method may alleviate patients' initial apprehensions. Anchoring involves using a more well-known concept as a point of reference for introducing or comparing a newer concept. A classic example would be using insulin as an anchor for biologics. In this instance, we would counsel patients on how both medications are delivered as injections. However, while insulin requires daily injections, biologics typically require less frequent injections [2]. If a patient is started on a biologic and you suspect low adherence, you may offer an office visit to administer the initial injection(s) until the patient becomes more familiar with the medication.

REFERENCES

[1]   Lewis DJ, Feldman SR. Practical Ways to Improve Patient Adherence. Create Space Independent Publishing Platform; c. Clinical Studies on Adherence 2017; pp. 27-40.

[2]   Lewis DJ, Feldman SR. Practical Ways to Improve Patient Adherence. Create Space Independent Publishing Platform; c. Anchoring 2017; pp. 110-4.

CHAPTER 6

Moisturizer Pearls

Mohammad Reza Namazi[1,*]

¹ Shiraz University of Medical Sciences and Dr. Namazi Skin and Hair Clinic, Shiraz, Iran

Moisturizers are used to relieve skin dryness, disguise fine wrinkles, and as a base for make-up.

Manufactured moisturizer creams contain emulsifiers to stabilize the emulsion. Emulsifiers derange the stratum corneum lipid structure, causing enhanced transepidermal water loss with resultant skin dryness, itchiness, irritation, and redness. You may have had patients saying: "I use my moisturizer, but my skin still feels dry!". Moreover, the preservatives and fragrances in scented products can further irritate the damaged skin. For these reasons, many commercial creams are not tolerated by people with sensitive skin. Therefore, some clinicians prefer emulsifier-free creams, which instead of emulsifiers, contain cell membrane components similar to the barrier layers of the skin [1].

Prescribing ointments which do not contain emulsifiers and freshly prepared compound moisturizers are other options.

Provided are the formulations of some compound emollients from the author's experience, which can be freshly made by your local pharmacist:

5% glycerin in eucerin is a simple, cheap and good moisturizer.

5-10% urea + 2% LA + 5% glycerin + 5% N/S in eucerin is a stronger moisturizer. (LA: Lactic Acid; N/S: Normal Saline). 20% dexpanthenol cream 5% and 2% nicotinamide powder may be added to this formula (In this case, 20% of the compound would be composed of dexpanthenol cream 5%, therefore having 1% dexpanthenol. This compound contains a small amount of the emulsifiers present in the dexpanthenol cream, which is very unlikely to irritate the skin):

* **Corresponding author Mohammad Reza Namazi:** Shiraz University of Medical Sciences and Dr. Namazi Skin and Hair Clinic, Shiraz, Iran; E-mail: rezanamazi12@yahoo.com

5-10% urea + 2% LA + 5% glycerin + 20% dexpanthenol cream + 2% nicotinamide + 5% N/S in eucerin. Description of the ingredients of the above compounds:

• Glycerin is a humectant (water-retaining substance). It attracts water from the environment into the skin. In 5% concentration, it can also be compounded with petrolatum (Vaseline).

• Eucerin is a good base for both water- and oil-soluble ingredients. Therefore, when mixing a cream (mixture of oil and water) with an ointment, pharmacists add some eucerin to the mixture to stabilize it to prevent it from becoming biphasic.

• Urea is a humectant and penetration enhancer (increases the penetration of other agents), and also improves the skin barrier function by inducing the expression of cornified envelope proteins. Urea at 2-10% concentrations causes moisturisation and optimises skin barrier function, at 10-30% causes moisturisation and keratolysis, and at ≥ 30% exerts keratolysis and debridement of necrotic tissues, such as callosities [2].

Urea is highly water soluble. Therefore, petroleum jelly (petrolatum) is not a good vehicle for it, while eucerin is. Urea should be used at 1-3% concentrations in young children to prevent irritation.

• Lactic acid is a humectant and keratolytic that induces ceramide production by keratinocytes, thus improving barrier function [3]. It is a fluid and can be mixed with both water and alcohol.

• Nicotinamide (Niacinamide) has anti-inflammatory, anti-oxidant, ceramide synthesis increment, antigen-induced lymphocyte transformation inhibition, and mast cell stabilising effects. Therefore, this agent can be a useful addition to the anti-atopic dermatitis armamentarium [4].

• Pantothenic acid is essential for normal epithelial function. Topical dexpanthenol is anti-inflammatory, acts like a moisturizer, improves stratum corneum hydration, and accelerates re-epithelization. Usually, the topical administration of dexpanthenol preparations is well tolerated, with minimal risk of skin irritation or sensitisation. Moreover, activation of fibroblast proliferation, which is of relevance in wound healing, has been observed both *in vitro* and *in vivo* with dexpanthenol [5].

Emulsifying ointment is a mixture of paraffin oils and is used to moisturise the skin. It contains sodium lauryl sulphate as well, which can irritate the skin.

Paraffin is a by-product of the petrochemical industry. It has an unpleasant smell and is not preferable to use, so manufacturers add preservatives and fragrances to it, which can irritate sensitive skin. Emulsifying ointments can catch fire when present on clothes because they contain paraffin oils. The patient should keep away from open fires and flames, *e.g.*, fireplaces [6].

As a single agent, petrolatum (petroleum jelly, white petrolatum, soft paraffin) is a good moisturizer. Vaseline is its well-known American brand. Petrolatum is flammable only when heated to liquid and only the fumes will light, not the liquid itself. It is colorless (or of a pale yellow color when not highly distilled) and devoid of taste and smell when pure.

Allergic reactions to petrolatum itself are very rare [7], but scented products can irritate sensitive skin. Petrolatum is incompatible with latex products and can cause condom breakage.

If you do not want to prescribe a freshly prepared compound moisturizer, QV cream and the greasier QV intensive moisturizer are excellent moisturizers, even for sensitive skin. QV intensive moisturizer cleanser is an excellent cleanser for dry, sensitive skin.

Moisturizers coming from a pump are usually too thin and not good.

Bath oils can be used for moisturising the body, especially for acne-prone patients, if specific emollients for acne-prone skin are not available.

Advise the patients not to rub the moisturizers on the skin, as this can further disturb the skin barrier.

The order of application of emollients and steroids does not matter in the treatment of atopic dermatitis [8]. Given that the application of tacrolimus on irritated skin can cause a burning sensation, prior application of an emollient can resolve this problem, as tacrolimus dissolves in the emollient and gradually comes into contact with the skin and penetrates it.

REFERENCES

[1]   International Association for Applied Corneotherapy. Available from: https://corneotherapy.org/articles/emulsifiers-in-skin-care

[2]   Piquero-Casals J, Morgado-Carrasco D, Granger C, Trullàs C, Jesús-Silva A, Krutmann J. Urea in dermatology: A review of its emollient, moisturizing, keratolytic, skin barrier enhancing and antimicrobial properties. Dermatol Ther 2021; 11(6): 1905-15.
[http://dx.doi.org/10.1007/s13555-021-00611-y] [PMID: 34596890]

[3]   Burkhart CG, Katz KA. Other topical medications. In: Goldsmith LA, Katz SI, Gilchrest BA, Paller AS, Leffell AJ, Wolf K, Eds. Other topican medications In: Fitzpatrick's Dermatology in General Medicine. 8th ed. USA: McGraw-Hill 2012; pp. 2697-707.

[4] Namazi MR. Nicotinamide as a potential addition to the anti-atopic dermatitis armamentarium. Int Immunopharmacol 2004; 4(6): 709-12.
[http://dx.doi.org/10.1016/j.intimp.2003.11.008] [PMID: 15135312]

[5] Ebner F, Heller A, Rippke F, Tausch I. Topical use of dexpanthenol in skin disorders. Am J Clin Dermatol 2002; 3(6): 427-33.
[http://dx.doi.org/10.2165/00128071-200203060-00005] [PMID: 12113650]

[6] Health Navigator Website. Emulsifying ointment. Available from: https://www.healthnavigator.org.nz/medicines/e/emulsifying-ointment/

[7] Willkinson SM, Beck MH. Contact dermatitis: Allergic.Rook's Textbook of Dermatology. 8th ed. Singapore: Wiley-Blackwell 2010; p. 2685.
[http://dx.doi.org/10.1002/9781444317633.ch25]

[8] Ng SY, Begum S, Chong SY. Does order of application of emollient and topical corticosteroids make a difference in the severity of atopic eczema in children? Pediatr Dermatol 2016; 33(2): 160-4.
[http://dx.doi.org/10.1111/pde.12758] [PMID: 26856694]

CHAPTER 7

How to Make an Oily Calamine Compound Which Does Not Dry the Skin?

Mohammad Reza Namazi[1,*]

[1] *Shiraz University of Medical Sciences and Dr. Namazi Skin and Hair Clinic, Shiraz, Iran*

Calamine is zinc oxide plus a very small amount of ferric oxide. It is produced with additional ingredients, such as phenol [1, 2].

Calamine lotion/cream is used for relieving itch, *e.g.*, from that of an insect bite, but it dries the skin, which is undesirable if the skin is already xerotic.

Prescribe the following compound for making 'oily calamine' which does not dry the skin:

5% glycerin in calamine cream/lotion.

REFERENCES

[1]   Joy N. Calamine lotion J Skin Sex Transm Dis 2022; 4: 83-6.

[2]   Dermnet. Pruritus. Available from: https://dermnetnz.org/topics/pruritus (Accessed: 31/12/2021).

* **Corresponding author Mohammad Reza Namazi:** Shiraz University of Medical Sciences and Dr. Namazi Skin and Hair Clinic, Shiraz, Iran; E-mail: rezanamazi12@yahoo.com

CHAPTER 8

How to Make Strong Topical Anti-Itch Compounds?

Mohammad Reza Namazi[1,*]

¹ Shiraz University of Medical Sciences and Dr. Namazi Skin and Hair Clinic, Shiraz, Iran

Prescribing a potent topical anti-pruritic compound for extremely itchy skin conditions is sometimes needed. Below, you will find useful information regarding topical anti-itch agents and compounds:

-Phenol (0.5% to 2%) is antipruritic due to its anesthetic effect. It should be avoided in pregnancy.

-Menthol and camphor are of plant origin and exert antipruritic effects by acting at transient receptor potential channels (TRP channels) [1]. Menthol is highly lipid soluble and may be used at up to 2% concentration, but many patients dislike concentrations more than 0.5% due to its unpleasant odor.

-Calamine lotion contains phenol, which cools the skin [2]. In the author's experience, 0.5% menthol and 0.5% camphor can be added to it to make a stronger anti-pruritic topical: 0.5% menthol + 0.5% camphor in calamine cream/lotion.

-0.5% menthol + 5% glycerin in calamine cream/lotion has a stronger anti-itch effect than calamine per se and does not dry the skin.

-0.5% menthol, 0.5% camphor and 0.5% phenol can be added to emollients to have an additional anti-itch effect:

0.5% menthol + 0.5% phenol + 0.5% camphor + 5% glycerin in eucerin.

-Another anti-itch formula is 0.5% menthol + 0.5% phenol + 0.5% camphor in cold cream. Cold cream is an oil-in-water emulsion characterized by rapid evaporation of water, giving a cooling effect that alleviates the itch sensation.

* **Corresponding author Mohammad Reza Namazi:** Shiraz University of Medical Sciences and Dr. Namazi Skin and Hair Clinic, Shiraz, Iran; E-mail: rezanamazi12@yahoo.com

REFERENCES

[1]   Metz M, Staubach P. Itch management: Topical agents. Curr Probl Dermatol 2016; 50: 40-5.
      [http://dx.doi.org/10.1159/000446040] [PMID: 27578070]

[2]   Dermnet. Pruritus. Available from: https://dermnetnz.org/topics/pruritus (Accessed 31/12/2021).

CHAPTER 9

Topical Steroids and Steroid Vehicles: Some Pearls

Mohammad Reza Namazi[1,*]

[1] *Shiraz University of Medical Sciences and Dr. Namazi Skin and Hair Clinic, Shiraz, Iran*

The potency of steroids may differ based on their vehicles.

Ointments offer more lubrication and occlusion than other preparations and are beneficial for dry or thick hyperkeratotic lesions. Their occlusive property also enhances the penetration of corticosteroids [1].

Creams are a mixture of water suspended in oil. Absorbance into the skin makes them cosmetically desirable. Creams are generally less potent than ointments of the same medication, and they usually have preservatives, which can induce irritation, stinging, and allergic reactions. Acute exudative inflammation responds better to creams due to their drying effect. Additionally, creams are useful in intertriginous areas where ointments may not be used. However, creams do not offer the same degree of occlusion as the ointments.

Creams should not be used on dry dermatitis areas, as they can cause irritation due to their emulsifiers, thus ointments are preferred [1].

Lotions and gels are the least oily and occlusive of all the topical vehicles. Lotions contain alcohol, which dries oozing lesions. Gels possess a jelly-like consistency and are useful for exudating lesions. Gels dry rapidly and can be applied on the scalp or other hairy areas without causing matting [1].

Using a topical steroid following a shower/bath enhances the steroid efficacy, as hydration generally promotes steroid penetration. Ordinary plastic dressings also increase the steroid penetration by severalfold [1].

Some dermatologists prescribe 2% lactic acid and 2% salicylic acid compounded with steroids to increase steroid penetration (*e.g.*, 2% salicylic acid + 2% lactic acid in clobestasol, or 2% salicylic acid + 2% lactic acid + 40% clobestasol in petrolatum). Salicylic and lactic acids at these low concentrations do not cause

* **Corresponding author Mohammad Reza Namazi:** Shiraz University of Medical Sciences and Dr. Namazi Skin and Hair Clinic, Shiraz, Iran; E-mail: rezanamazi12@yahoo.com

irritation, even in acute disease stages. As salicylic acid and lactic acid work on different layers of the horny layer to exert their keratolytic actions, their combination can increase the penetration of steroids significantly. Lactic acid is available as a fluid, while salicylic acid is in the form of powder. A common mistake is the absolute avoidance of using potent steroids, like clobetasol, for treating severe dermatoses in areas having thin skin, such as the face and intertriginous areas. Potent steroids can be used for a few days to control acute dermatoses without causing atrophy. The treatment can then be switched to other topicals, like calcineurin inhibitors or less atrophogenic steroids, such as mometasone. This dramatically enhances patient's adherence and comfort. Note that the use of calcineurin inhibitors for acute dermatoses can irritate the skin or cause a burning sensation. Using topical clobetasol on the lids for a few days does not cause any problem. Another common mistake is to prescribe topical hydrocortisone for dermatoses in children. It is usually ineffective because of its very low potency. Prescribing a topical compound containing diluted potent steroids, *e.g.*, 20% mometasone ointment 0.1% in petrolatum, or a calcineurin inhibitor, like pimecrolimus or tacrolimus, is a much better option. Topical hydrocortisone can be effective against mild dermatoses in the periocular area.

Mometasone furoate is a potent steroid having low risk of local and systemic adverse effects. It can be applied just once daily, as the effectiveness of mometasone furoate 0.1% ointment, cream and lotion applied once per day was found to be equal to or more than that of several other very potent steroids with a similar formulation requiring twice or thrice daily application [2].

In the author's experience, tacrolimus BD (mane and nocte) plus mometasone or clobetasol QD (at midday) rapidly controls very severe dermatoses. However, no clinical trial is available on this suggestion.

In the author's experience, intralesional steroids can resolve idiopathic localized chronic pruritus unresponsive to other measures.

REFERENCES

[1]   Ference JD, Last AR. Choosing topical corticosteroids. Am Fam Physician 2009; 79(2): 135-40.
       [PMID: 19178066]

[2]   Spada F, Barnes TM, Greive KA. Comparative safety and efficacy of topical mometasone furoate with
       other topical corticosteroids. Australas J Dermatol 2018; 59(3): 168-74.
       [http://dx.doi.org/10.1111/ajd.12762] [PMID: 29411351]

CHAPTER 10

Steroids: Some Pearls

Mohammad Reza Namazi[1,*]

[1] *Shiraz University of Medical Sciences and Dr. Namazi Skin and Hair Clinic, Shiraz, Iran*

Steroids are one of the most commonly used drugs in dermatology. Some pearls on these agents are presented below:

Regarding the use of prednisolone in pregnancy, Rook's Textbook of Dermatology mentions that for severe pemphigoid gestationis, 40–80 mg/d of prednisolone can be used. Prednisolone dosage is usually decreased fairly rapidly to a much lower maintenance dose after controlling the disease activity. Systemic steroids do not seem to adversely affect pregnancy outcomes [1]. However, some adverse effects are mentioned in other publications.

-Topical steroids can cause congenital defects in animals if used in large amounts, under occlusion, or for long duration. They have not demonstrated to do so in humans and are classified by the FDA as pregnancy category C.

-The excretion of topical steroids in breast milk is uncertain. As a precaution, topical steroids should be applied to the breasts instantly after nursing to allow maximal time before the next feeding [2].

The American Academy of Pediatrics has determined that prednisolone therapy is compatible with breastfeeding, though it is best to delay it for 4 hours after taking the drug [3]. Systemic effects of prednisolone in infants are unlikely with maternal doses less than 40 mg/d [4].

Taking prednisolone in childhood can slow down the child's growth, however, after discontinuation, catch-up is anticipated, provided that adolescence is not completed. For this reason, steroids should be avoided, if possible, during the period of rapid growth in adolescence, *i.e.*, 11 years in girls and 13 years in boys [5]. Some references also recommend avoidance of steroids during childhood spurt, *i.e.*, first 2 years. Therefore, growth monitoring every 3-6 months is warranted [3, 6].

---

[*] **Corresponding author Mohammad Reza Namazi:** Shiraz University of Medical Sciences and Dr. Namazi Skin and Hair Clinic, Shiraz, Iran; E-mail: rezanamazi12@yahoo.com

Short courses of systemic steroids can be given to HIV patients since no significant effects on CD4 counts are noted [6].

Prednisolone does not need any adjustment in renal failure [7].

Prednisone tapering can be done as follows:

• Doses > 40 mg/day – taper by 10 mg/week to 40 mg/d, which is maintained for 1 week.

• 40 mg/day – taper by 5 mg/week to 20 mg/d, which is maintained for 1 week.

• 20 mg/day – taper by 2.5 mg/week to 5 mg/d, which is maintained for 1 week.

• 5 mg/day – taper by 1 mg/week until discontinuation [8].

REFERENCES

[1]   Wojnarowska F, Venning VA. Immunobullous Diseases.Rook's Textbook of Dermatology. 8th ed. Singapore: Wiley-Blackwell 2010; p. 45.
      [http://dx.doi.org/10.1002/9781444317633.ch40]

[2]   Ference JD, Last AR. Choosing topical corticosteroids. Am Fam Physician 2009; 79(2): 135-40.
      [PMID: 19178066]

[3]   Jackson S, Gilchrist H, Nesbitt LT Jr. Update on the dermatologic use of systemic glucocorticosteroids. Dermatol Ther 2007; 20(4): 187-205.
      [http://dx.doi.org/10.1111/j.1529-8019.2007.00133.x] [PMID: 17970885]

[4]   Wakelin SH. Handbook of Systemic Drug Treatment in Dermatology. 1st ed. London: Manson Publishing Ltd. 2002; p. 220.
      [http://dx.doi.org/10.1201/b16367]

[5]   Ryu RJ, Easterling TR, Caritis SN, Venkataramanan R, Umans JG, Ahmed MS, Clark S, Kantrowitz-Gordon I, Hays K, Bennett B, Honaker MT, Thummel KE, Shen DD, Hebert MF. Prednisone Pharmacokinetics During Pregnancy and Lactation. J Clin Pharmacol. 2018 Sep;58(9):1223-1232.
      [http://dx.doi.org/10.1002/jcph.1122] [PMID: 29733485]

[6]   Ryu RJ, Easterling TR, Caritis SN, Venkataramanan R, Umans JG, Ahmed MS, Clark S, Kantrowitz-Gordon I, Hays K, Bennett B, Honaker MT, Thummel KE, Shen DD, Hebert MF. Prednisone Pharmacokinetics During Pregnancy and Lactation. J Clin Pharmacol. 2018 Sep; 58(9): 1223-1232. Epub 2018 May 7.
      [http://dx.doi.org/10.1002/jcph.1122] [PMID: 29733485] [PMCID: PMC6310475]

[7]   Ryu RJ, Easterling TR, Caritis SN, *et al.* Prednisone Pharmacokinetics During Pregnancy and Lactation J Clin Pharmacol 2018 Sep; 58(9): 1223-32.
      [http://dx.doi.org/10.1002/jcph.1122] [PMID: 29733485]

[8]   Caplan A, Fett N, Rosenbach M, Werth VP, Micheletti RG. Prevention and management of glucocorticoid-induced side effects: A comprehensive review. J Am Acad Dermatol 2017; 76(2): 201-7.
      [http://dx.doi.org/10.1016/j.jaad.2016.02.1241] [PMID: 28088991]

CHAPTER 11

Steroid Comparison Table

Mohammad Reza Namazi[1,*]

[1] Shiraz University of Medical Sciences and Dr. Namazi Skin and Hair Clinic, Shiraz, Iran

Strangely, the steroid comparison table (Table **1**), while being useful, is missing from some major textbooks.

Table 1. Comparison of steroids with respect to anti-inflammatory and mineralocorticoid effects and the duration of the effect on Hypothalamic-Pituitary-Adrenal Axis (HPA) (From references 1 and 2, with adaptations). HPA: Hypothalamic-Pituitary-Adrenal Axis; S: Short-acting, I: Intermediate acting, L: Long-acting.

Active Principle	Equivalent Anti – inflammatory Dose*	Mineralocorticoid Effect	Duration of Effect on HPA
Hydrocortisone	20 mg	0.8	12 (S)
Prednisone	5 mg	0.8	12-36 (I)
Prednisolone	5 mg	0.8	12-36 (I)
Methylprednisolone	4 mg	0.5	12-36 (I)
Triamcinolone	4 mg	0	12-36 (I)
Betamethasone	0.8 mg	0	>48 (L)
Dexamethasone	0.8 mg	0	>48 (L)

* The anti-inflammatory effect corresponds to the glucocorticoid effect.

Note that the related figures for dexamethasone and betamethasone vary slightly in different references. Moreover, these dose relationships only apply to oral or intravenous administration, and glucocorticoid potencies may differ greatly following intramuscular administration.

Memorising the steroid equivalent doses may not be easy. A good mnemonic is MPH (Master of Public Health), where M is methylprednisolone (4), P is prednisolone (5) and H is hydrocortisone (20) [4 × 5 = 20]. To know the whole, you would just need to memorise that triamcinolone is equipotent with methyl-

*Corresponding author Mohammad Reza Namazi:** Shiraz University of Medical Sciences and Dr. Namazi Skin and Hair Clinic, Shiraz, Iran; E-mail: rezanamazi12@yahoo.com

prednisolone and that both dexamethasone and betamethasone have comparable equivalent doses (0.8).

According to this table, if you like to replace a hospitalized patient's dexamethasone dosed at 12 mg/d with prednisolone, you need to prescribe prednisolone at 75 mg/d to have nearly the same anti-inflammatory effect. Also, the table shows that for hypertensive patients, betamethasone, triamcinolone and dexamethasone are better choices.

As hydrocortisone has much less glucocorticoid effect than other steroids, it can be beneficial for hospitalized diabetic patients, but it produces a strong mineralocorticoid effect.

REFERENCES

[1]   MD+Calc. Available from: https://www.mdcalc.com/calc/2040/steroid-conversion-calculator (Accessed: 12/15/2022).

[2]   Key V. Available from: https://veteriankey.com/glucocorticoids-and-mineralocorticoids/ (Accessed: 12/7/2022).

CHAPTER 12

Pulse Steroid Therapy

Mohammad Reza Namazi[1,*]

[1] *Shiraz University of Medical Sciences and Dr. Namazi Skin and Hair Clinic, Shiraz, Iran*

Pulse Steroid Therapy (PST) is the parenteral administration of glucocorticoids in short bursts of supra pharmacological doses. Unfortunately, this very useful therapeutic approach seems to be underutilised by dermatologists.

-Some examples of dermatologic conditions in which PST is used successfully include toxic epidermal necrolysis, erythema multiforme major, pyoderma gangrenosum, pemphigus, bullous pemphigoid, epidermolysis bullosa aquisita, erythroderma, and generalized lichen planus [1].

-Advantages of PST include rapid response and avoidance of prolonged high-dose oral corticosteroids [1].

For pulse therapy, methylprednisolone is given in doses of 0.5 to 1 g dissolved in 200 ml of 5% dextrose over 2 hours daily for 1-5 days (20–30 mg/kg/d, maximum dose of 1 g/d) [2]. A 1 g dose of methylprednisolone has an anti-inflammatory effect equal to about 1250 mg of prednisolone (250 prednisolone 5 mg tablets or 25 prednisolone 50 mg tablets). Low-dose oral corticosteroids or other immunosuppressive agents are used as maintenance therapy once a remission is achieved, with additional courses given one to several weeks later for recalcitrant disease or prevention of recurrence [1].

Some references advise that cardiac monitoring is required for possible arrhythmias [2]. These recommendations are based on case reports of adverse cardiovascular effects, including sudden death of patients treated with PST for nondermatologic conditions. Many specialists in non-dermatology fields with years of experience with PST do not intensively monitor all patients who receive PST and may administer PST on an outpatient basis.

---

* **Corresponding author Mohammad Reza Namazi:** Shiraz University of Medical Sciences and Dr. Namazi Skin and Hair Clinic, Shiraz, Iran; E-mail: rezanamazi12@yahoo.com

Some rheumatologists who are reluctant to administer PST in the outpatient setting state that oral pulse dosing, if established to be of equal efficacy, would allow outpatient administration [1].

A study on a single intravenous methylprednisolone 30 mg/kg administered over 10 minutes to healthy volunteers showed no significant alterations in blood sugar, electrolytes, liver and renal function tests, vital signs and blood pressure, ECG and EEG, with preservation of the ability of the adrenal gland to respond to ACTH stimulation test [3]. However, continuous cardiac monitoring is clearly indicated for patients with cardiac or renal disease. Furosemide administration before PST has been proposed as a possible factor in sudden death. Daily monitoring of electrolytes before infusion and for 24 hours afterward is indicated in patients with cardiac disease, renal disease, and in those with compromised skin integrity (i.e., pemphigus, toxic epidermal necrolysis, and erythroderma) who may likewise be predisposed to electrolyte shifts. Otherwise, outpatient administration of PST may not be unsafe but cannot be firmly recommended without a prospective trial confirming its safety [1].

If PST is given rapidly, sudden death may occur. Acute electrolyte shifts causing cardiac problems can be prevented by slow infusion over 2 hours. A high potassium diet can be helpful [3].

Patient's blood pressure should be monitored during pulse therapy [3].

In hypertensive patients, dexamethasone pulse therapy may be considered, given dexamethasone's lack of mineralocorticoid effect, however dexamethasone has a stronger glucocorticoid effect than methylprednisolone (See the Steroid Comparison Table in the previous chapter).

Methylprednisolone, 2 mg/kg/day in divided doses every 6-8 hours, can also be used to control severe diseases [3].

REFERENCES

[1]   White KP, Driscoll MS, Rothe MJ, Grant-Kels JM. Severe adverse cardiovascular effects of pulse steroid therapy: Is continuous cardiac monitoring necessary? J Am Acad Dermatol 1994; 30(5): 768-73.
       [http://dx.doi.org/10.1016/S0190-9622(08)81508-3] [PMID: 8176017]

[2]   Novak E, Stubbs SS, Seckman CE, Hearron MS. Effects of a single large intravenous dose of methylprednisolone sodium succinate. Clin Pharmacol Ther 1970; 11(5): 711-7.
       [http://dx.doi.org/10.1002/cpt1970115711] [PMID: 4917091]

[3]   Jackson S, Gilchrist H, Nesbitt LT Jr. Update on the dermatologic use of systemic glucocorticosteroids. Dermatol Ther 2007; 20(4): 187-205.
       [http://dx.doi.org/10.1111/j.1529-8019.2007.00133.x] [PMID: 17970885]

CHAPTER 13

Intradermal Triamcinolone Injection

Mohammad Reza Namazi[1,*]

[1] *Shiraz University of Medical Sciences and Dr. Namazi Skin and Hair Clinic, Shiraz, Iran*

Intradermal triamcinolone injection is the mainstay of treatment of focal alopecia areata.

A meta-analysis shows that the rates of hair regrowth are comparable in 5 mg/ml and 10 mg/ml concentrations, while lower regrowth rates are seen in lower concentrations. Given the risk-benefit ratio, 5 mg/ml concentration may offer the greatest benefit to these patients [1].

The excipients of different triamcinolone ampoules are not observed to be the same and the injectable triamcinolone made in some countries, such as Iran, does not mix well with lidocaine and makes a precipitate. The brochure of this kind of triamcinolone ampoule also clearly states that it should not be injected into the skin. Injection of this kind of triamcinolone, *e.g.*, for treating alopecia areata, can cause skin atrophy as the injected mixture is not uniform. In the peri-ocular area, including brows, it can cause blindness by clogging ocular vessels. Kenacort is a sort of triamcinolone that is mixed well with lidocaine. If not available, you can use hydrocortisone, betamethasone or dexamethasone ampoules (See the Steroid Comparison Table in this book). 25 mg hydrocortisone is equipotent with 5 mg triamcinolone (See the Steroid Comparison Table, Chapter 11). Therefore, if you would like to inject intralesional hydrocortisone into a patient's eyebrow instead of triamcinolone 5 mg/ml, you would need to produce hydrocortisone at 25 mg/ml concentration. As a hydrocortisone vial contains 100 mg of hydrocortisone, you can add 2cc lidocaine to the vial, then pull up 0.5 cc of the solution into a 1 cc syringe and fill the rest of the syringe with lidocaine. Now, you have 1 cc of hydrocortisone at 25 mg/ml concentration.

---

* **Corresponding author Mohammad Reza Namazi:** Shiraz University of Medical Sciences and Dr. Namazi Skin and Hair Clinic, Shiraz, Iran; E-mail: rezanamazi12@yahoo.com

REFERENCE

[1] Yee BE, Tong Y, Goldenberg A, Hata T. Efficacy of different concentrations of intralesional triamcinolone acetonide for alopecia areata: A systematic review and meta-analysis. J Am Acad Dermatol 2020; 82(4): 1018-21.
[http://dx.doi.org/10.1016/j.jaad.2019.11.066] [PMID: 31843657]

CHAPTER 14

Increasing the Efficacy of Intravenous N-acetylcysteine

Mohammad Reza Namazi[1,*]

[1] *Shiraz University of Medical Sciences and Dr. Namazi Skin and Hair Clinic, Shiraz, Iran*

Intravenous N-acetylcysteine (NAC) has been reported to be effective in severe adverse cutaneous drug reactions, probably by increasing intracellular glutathione levels, which has a detoxifying action [1]. NAC may be especially useful in patients with reduced intracellular glutathione levels, such as HIV-positive and G6PD-deficient patients.

An important point is that NAC is acidic due to its carboxyl group and the absence of a free amino group [2]. This means that in the basic PH of blood, it ionizes and cannot penetrate the cell membranes well. Therefore, to increase its efficacy, it is advisable to induce respiratory acidosis by asking the patient to breathe in a plastic bag from time to time during drug administration.

REFERENCES

[1]   Hasan MJ, Rabbani R. Intravenous N-acetylcysteine in severe cutaneous drug reaction treatment: A case series. SAGE Open Med Case Rep 2020; 20.

[2]   Pedre B, Barayeu U, Ezeriņa D, Dick TP. The mechanism of action of N-acetylcysteine (NAC): The emerging role of H_2S and sulfane sulfur species. Pharmacol Ther 2021; 228: 107916.
[http://dx.doi.org/10.1016/j.pharmthera.2021.107916] [PMID: 34171332]

[*] **Corresponding author Mohammad Reza Namazi:** Shiraz University of Medical Sciences and Dr. Namazi Skin and Hair Clinic, Shiraz, Iran; E-mail: rezanamazi12@yahoo.com

CHAPTER 15

Postherpetic Neuralgia: Pearls

Mohammad Reza Namazi[1,*]

[1] *Shiraz University of Medical Sciences and Dr. Namazi Skin and Hair Clinic, Shiraz, Iran*

Post-herpetic neuralgia (PHN) is often very difficult to treat. Treatments include topical lidocaine (often considered first-line therapy), topical capsaicin, gabapentin, pregabalin and tricyclic anti-depressants (TCA) [1].

Treating PHN in the elderly with TCA poses some problems. Glaucoma, benign prostatic hyperplasia, memory problems and heart rhythm disorders are more common in the elderly. These problems, as well as constipation, can be exacerbated by drugs having anti-cholinergic effects, such as TCA.

Desipramine, followed by nortriptyline, has the lowest anticholinergic side effects among the TCA. Amitryptiline and doxepine have the strongest anticholinergic effects [2]. Therefore, desipramine is the best TCA for managing postherpetic neuralgia in the elderly.

Sometimes, postherpetic neuralgia presents as pruritus. Many dermatologists manage this condition with anti-histamines. However, this itch is caused by neuropathy, not by the excessive release of histamine, and cannot be alleviated by anti-histamines.

According to some references, haloperidol (3×0.5-1 mg per day) is useful against burning dysesthesia, while valproic acid (3×100 mg per day, maximum 4×600 mg) is useful against intermittent lancinating pain.

There is currently some evidence for the therapeutic effect of vitamin B12 in the treatment of post-herpetic neuralgia (level II evidence). Vitamin B12 can decrease neuropathic pain by enhancing myelination and nerve regeneration, as well as, decreasing ectopic nerve firing [3]. In rats, a combination of vitamin B12 and vitamin E acetate improved sciatic nerve crush injury, which may be applicable to the treatment of postherpetic neuralgia. Curcumin and alpha-lipoic acid also have neuronal regeneration capacity [4].

* **Corresponding author Mohammad Reza Namazi:** Shiraz University of Medical Sciences and Dr. Namazi Skin and Hair Clinic, Shiraz, Iran; E-mail: rezanamazi12@yahoo.com

In zoster patients, prednisone reduces acute pain; however, it does not reduce the risk of PHN [1].

Should anti-virals be initiated if a patient who has not taken anti-virals comes with postherpetic neuralgia? Although anti-virals therapy reduces acute pain associated with zoster, it has not been shown to reliably reduce the risk of PHN, nor is it recommended for the treatment of established PHN [1]. However, varicella and zoster, especially ophthalmic zoster, are risk factors for stroke, particularly in individuals who develop zoster under 40 years of age. Anti-viral therapy may decrease this risk. Therefore, starting anti-virals in the questioned situation seems wise [5]. It is also apt to evaluate these patients for stroke risk factors, such as hypertension.

REFERENCES

[1]   Gershon AA, Breuer J, Cohen JI, *et al.* Varicella zoster virus infection. Nat Rev Dis Primers 2015; 1(1): 15016.
        [http://dx.doi.org/10.1038/nrdp.2015.16] [PMID: 27188665]

[2]   Namazi MR. Prescribing cyclic antidepressants for vitiligo patients: Which agents are superior, which are not? Psychother Psychosom 2003; 72(6): 361-2.
        [http://dx.doi.org/10.1159/000073036] [PMID: 14526142]

[3]   Julian T, Syeed R, Glascow N, Angelopoulou E, Zis P. B12 as a treatment for peripheral neuropathic pain: A systematic review. Nutrients 2020; 12(8): 2221.
        [http://dx.doi.org/10.3390/nu12082221] [PMID: 32722436]

[4]   Abushukur Y, Knackstedt R. The impact of supplements on recovery after peripheral nerve injury: A review of the literature. Cureus 2022; 14(5): 25135.
        [http://dx.doi.org/10.7759/cureus.25135] [PMID: 35733475]

[5]   Amlie-Lefond C, Gilden D. Varicella zoster virus: A common cause of stroke in children and adults. J Stroke Cerebrovasc Dis 2016; 25(7): 1561-9.
        [http://dx.doi.org/10.1016/j.jstrokecerebrovasdis.2016.03.052] [PMID: 27138380]

CHAPTER 16

An Important Point in Intravenous Acyclovir Administration

Mohammad Reza Namazi[1,*]

[1] *Shiraz University of Medical Sciences and Dr. Namazi Skin and Hair Clinic, Shiraz, Iran*

Intravenously administered acyclovir is generally used in zoster patients only if they are immunocompromised or are unable to take medications orally.

Intravenous (IV) acyclovir should be administered at a constant rate *via* IV infusion over 1 hour to prevent renal damage. It should be diluted in D5W or 0.9% NaCl solutions to a final concentration ≤ 7 mg/mL [1].

Some references stipulate hydrating the patient by giving 1.5 times maintenance hydration 1 hour before and also 1 hour after infusion [2].

Maintenance hydration is calculated as follows:

4 mL/kg/hr for the first 10 kg of body weight.

2 mL/kg/hr for the second 10 kg of body weight.

1 mL/g/hr for any kilogram of body mass above 20 kg.

REFERENCES

[1]   Taylor M, Gerriets V. Acyclovir. 2023 May 7. In: StatPearls [Internet]. Treasure Island (FL): StatPearls Publishing; 2024. PMID: 31194337

[2]   Cheo ED Outreach Website. Available from: https://outreach.cheo.on.ca/manual/1461# (Accessed 8/18/2022).

* **Corresponding author Mohammad Reza Namazi:** Shiraz University of Medical Sciences and Dr. Namazi Skin and Hair Clinic, Shiraz, Iran; E-mail: rezanamazi12@yahoo.com

CHAPTER 17

Genital Warts: Pearls

Mohammad Reza Namazi[1,*]

[1] *Shiraz University of Medical Sciences and Dr. Namazi Skin and Hair Clinic, Shiraz, Iran*

Genital warts are prevalent sexually-transmitted diseases caused by the Human Papilloma Virus (HPV).

It is mentioned in textbooks that condoms cannot provide protection against genital warts. This has caused the misconception that HPV can pass through condoms, however, it is untrue. HPV cannot pass through intact condoms, but it can infect the partner through contact with the areas not covered by the condom.

A frequently encountered question: "I have had only one partner for many years. Now that I have become HPV positive, does this mean that my partner has been having sex with another person?" Answer: About 5% of genital warts are not sexually transmitted [1]. Although rare, this hardy virus can possibly be transmitted in other ways, such as auto-inoculation (from hand to genital tract) [2]. In the author's experience, the use of a shared blade for waxing hair in unsanitary beauty saloons may transmit genital warts. Moreover, though the average incubation period of genital warts is 2 months to 2 years, its latency can extend to years or even a lifetime. During this time, the virus is always reproducing within cells with no manifestation of clinically apparent warts but can be transmitted by 70% of people in this phase through unprotected sex [1 - 3]. Therefore, it is also possible that the patient acquired the virus *via* sexual contact with another partner many, many years ago. Therefore, this patient may not only have not contracted the virus from his/ her current partner, but he/she may have even infected his/her current partner, however the partner could be in the incubation period or latency without having any discernible lesions. On the other hand, it is also possible that the patient has got HPV from his/her current partner, who is in the latent period. Many factors, such as a patient's immune status, determine the duration of the latency period.

90% of genital warts are caused by HPV types 6 and 11, which are low-risk subtypes and rarely cause cervical cancers. HPV genotypes 16, 18, 31, 33, and 35,

[*] **Corresponding author Mohammad Reza Namazi:** Shiraz University of Medical Sciences and Dr. Namazi Skin and Hair Clinic, Shiraz, Iran; E-mail: rezanamazi12@yahoo.com

considered high-risk, are infrequently found in genital warts but give rise to 99% of cervical cancers, with 70% caused by types 16 and 18 [3, 4]. Both high- and low-risk HPV subtypes have also been linked to verrucous carcinoma. Verrucous carcinoma is categorized into giant condyloma of Buschke and Löwenstein (anogenital area), oral florid papillomatosis (oral cavity), and carcinoma cuniculatum (palmoplantar surface) [3].

In very mild or subclinical cases, 3-5% acetic acid solution may help in wart visualization (acetowhite test) [3]. However, some believe that this test can be misleading and should not be used [1]. Conventional biopsy on suspected areas may also be misleading, as clear cells may be misidentified as koilocytes [1].

Oral sex carries little to no risk of getting or transmitting HIV; however, HPV and other sexually transmitted diseases (*i.e.*, syphilis, gonorrhea, and intestinal infections) can be transmitted. Genital warts may infrequently occur in the throat or mouth after oral sex with an infected individual. HPV can cause oral cancer [5]. HPV vaccine protects against oral infection caused by this virus [6].

Genital warts in children are often transmitted from parents. Transmission can occur during vaginal delivery in an asymptomatic woman, and the child's HPV infection can be latent for years before causing a wart. Also, in theory, a parent with a finger or hand wart can transmit HPV innocuously while bathing a child. Child abuse cannot be considered seriously if genital wart is the sole evidence of it [1].

The usual mode of HPV transmission to the newborn is through contact with infected maternal secretions during the passage through the birth canal, even in the absence of clinically evident lesions. However, the transmission can occur as a result of ascending infection from the vaginal canal following the premature rupture of amniotic membranes,from transplacental spread, or even from a sperm carrying latent HPV at the time of fertilization.

Laryngeal papillomatosis occurs due to perinatal transmission of HPV 6 or 11. The low risk of laryngeal papillomatosis and reports of its occurrence in children born by cesarean section (CS), along with the risks of CS, have resulted in the recommendation that the presence of genital warts cannot justify CS. In addition, no controlled studies have recommended that this rare possibility can be prevented by CS [7, 8]. CS is only indicated when extensive vaginal and/or introital warts block the birth canal. TCA, liquid nitrogen, laser ablation or electrosurgery can be employed for the treatment of external genital warts at any time during pregnancy, while the use of imiquimod is not approved. Podophyllin is potentially teratogenic and therefore contraindicated [7].

Most microbicides like benzalkonium chloride, N-9, octoxynol-9, as well as chlorhexidine are surfactants that destroy the envelopes of HSV-2 and HIV-1. However, these agents do not inactivate HPV, which is non-enveloped [9]. Chemical disinfectants used in healthcare settings, including glutaraldehyde, cannot destruct HPV, but bleach or autoclaving can [10]. Ultraviolet C can also destruct HPV.

The dermatologic literature recommends podophylline 25% in compound benzoin tincture applied weekly as an option for treating genital warts, with emphasis on the application performed by the physician, as podophylline can cause burn. However, this needs frequent visits by the patient which is usually difficult. In the author's experience, 15% podophylline in tincture of benzoin can be used by the patient if he/she is reliable. Ask the patient to apply it on the warts every other night using a cotton-tipped spatula for bigger warts and dental floss for tiny warts, being careful to avoid applying it to the surrounding normal skin. The patient can apply petrolatum or clear nail polish to the surrounding skin to ensure the medication does not come into contact with it, though this should not necessarily be done if the patient is very reliable and careful. The patient should be warned that excessive use can burn the skin and to wash the area immediately if it starts burning. He/she should wait for the topical to dry before wearing his/her underwear. The application should be temporarily discontinued if the wart ulcerates or becomes painful. It is usually effective in just a few weeks. Some patients who had applied it every day found it effective in less than two weeks without causing any problem.

Over-application of podophyllin on large condylomas can cause systemic side effects. As podophyllin is composed of some mutagens, purified podophyllotoxin preparations are produced but are not available widely [11].

For perianal warts, podophylline is effective but needs to be applied by a physician or a very reliable person, as there is a higher risk of irritation compared to the genital area. Imiquimod applied as a thin smear every other night before bedtime is very effective, but the effect may be seen after 2-3 weeks, thus it should be mentioned to the patient not to discontinue it prematurely.

Imiquimod does not cause graft rejection in organ transplant recipients [12]. Recurrence rates of warts are lower with imiquimod compared to podophyllin [13], and imiquimod is used for the treatment of intra-anal warts under anoscopy, including patients resistant to previous electrocautery, with a complete clearance rate of 70% at 28 weeks without severe adverse events [14]. Interestingly, when using imiquimod on actinic keratosis, inflammation of the apparently normal skin having subclinical actinic keratosis, *i.e.*, having very early pre-malignant alterations, is frequently noted, which results from the stimulation of the skin immune system to recognize and attack the abnormal cells [15]. If this effect is also proven to occur in genital warts, imiquimod can resolve latent HPV infection if used for treating genital warts. Imiquimod enhances Langerhans cell migration from the skin to draining lymph nodes, where Langerhans cells present antigens to CD4 T cells. A paper published in *Nature* reports Schiff base-forming drugs, including Vitamin B6, to enhance CD4 T cell activation by providing a costimulatory signal [16]. Vitamin B6, therefore, has the potential to enhance the therapeutic effect of imiquimod.

A novel pearl is that for giant warts in the groin and pubic regions, surgical resection is a very good option, as topical agents, cryotherapy, and intralesional interferon and bleomycine, usually fail. Any recurrence can then be treated with other options like cryotherapy, etc. This point strikingly contrasts with the popular belief that surgery is contraindicated in verrucae.

Genital verrucae frequently recur within 3 months after the completion of therapy. No cure for HPV is available, and treating visible warts does not necessarily decrease the transmission of the underlying HPV infection. However, in around 80% of HPV-positive cases, the infection resolves spontaneously within 18 to 24 months [13]. Cessation of smoking may help [13]. Theoretically, the use of immunity-enhancing drugs like zinc, selenium, and vitamin B6 may help.

Traditional theories posit that following the treatment, HPV remains in the body for the whole life. However, it is now believed that HPV may be either resolved or suppressed to low levels, which cannot be measured by polymerase chain reaction (PCR) tests. Age, smoking, and immunosuppression are some risk factors for the persistence of HPV infection [13].

Instillation of thiotepa can be effective for intraurethral lesions. Application of 5-fluorouracil 2-3 times daily is highly effective for urethral lesions in men, but rarely, it may cause urethral obstruction due to swelling. Intraurethral lesions are typically treated by a urologist [17]. Cystoscopy should be considered whenever the glans is involved and also in the presence of lower urinary tract symptoms or significant urethral symptoms. In patients having no symptoms, some experts have recommended waiting until the glans lesions have healed to prevent possible transfer of the virus into the urethra [13].

The CDC recommends conducting HPV vaccination at age 11 or 12 years, but it can be commenced as early as 9. For previously unvaccinated adults, CDC suggests vaccinations for 27 to 45-year-old individuals [17].

Gardasil provides protection against HPV types 6, 11, 16, and 18, offering 99% protection against genital warts (mainly caused by types 6, 11) and cervical cancer (mainly caused by types 16, 18). It is injected at baseline, 2 months, and 6 months. Cervarix provides protection against HPV types 16 and 18 and, therefore, cannot protect against genital warts (not useful for men). It is injected at baseline, 1 month, and 6 months [18].

REFERENCES

[1]   McNeil JS. Available from: https://cdn.mdedge.com/files/s3fs-public/issues/articles/70315_ main_2.pdf

[2]   Garland SM, Quinn MA. CHAPTER 11 How to manage and communicate with patients about HPV? Int J Gynaecol Obstet 2006; 94(S1) (1): S106-12.
        [http://dx.doi.org/10.1016/S0020-7292(07)60017-4] [PMID: 29644639]

[3]   Yanofsky VR, Patel RV, Goldenberg G. Genital warts: A comprehensive review. J Clin Aesthet Dermatol 2012; 5(6): 25-36.
        [PMID: 22768354]

[4]   Chen X, Li L, Lai Y, Liu Q, Yan J, Tang Y. Characteristics of human papillomaviruses infection in men with genital warts in Shanghai. Oncotarget 2016; 7(33): 53903-10.
        [http://dx.doi.org/10.18632/oncotarget.9708] [PMID: 27270315]

[5]   Available from: https://www.cdc.gov/std/healthcomm/stdfact-stdriskandoralsex.htm

[6]   Fiorillo L, Cervino G, Surace G, *et al.* Human Papilloma Virus: Current Knowledge and Focus on Oral Health. BioMed Res Int 2021; 2021: 1-10.
        [http://dx.doi.org/10.1155/2021/6631757] [PMID: 33623784]

[7]   Marfatia YS, Singhal P, Naswa S. Pregnancy and sexually transmitted viral infections. Indian J Sex Transm Dis 2009; 30(2): 71-8.
        [http://dx.doi.org/10.4103/0253-7184.62761] [PMID: 21938124]

[8]   Garland SM, Quinn MA. CHAPTER 11 How to manage and communicate with patients about HPV? Int J Gynaecol Obstet 2006; 94(S1) (1): 106-12.
        [http://dx.doi.org/10.1016/S0020-7292(07)60017-4] [PMID: 29644639]

[9]   Chilaka VN, Navti OB, Al Beloushi M, Ahmed B, Konje JC. Human papillomavirus (HPV) in pregnancy - An update. Eur J Obstet Gynecol Reprod Biol. 2021 Sep; 264: 340-348. Epub 2021 Jul 31.
        [http://dx.doi.org/10.1016/j.ejogrb.2021.07.053] [PMID: 34385080]

[10]   Meyers J, Ryndock E, Conway MJ, Meyers C, Robison R. Susceptibility of high-risk human papillomavirus type 16 to clinical disinfectants. J Antimicrob Chemother 2014; 69(6): 1546-50.
        [http://dx.doi.org/10.1093/jac/dku006] [PMID: 24500190]

[11]   Petersen CS, Weismann K. Quercetin and kaempherol: An argument against the use of podophyllin? Sex Transm Infect 1995; 71(2): 92-3.
        [http://dx.doi.org/10.1136/sti.71.2.92] [PMID: 7744421]

[12]   Ben M'barek L, Mebazaa A, Euvrard S, *et al.* 5% topical imiquimod tolerance in transplant recipients. Dermatology 2007; 215(2): 130-3.
        [http://dx.doi.org/10.1159/000104264] [PMID: 17684375]

[13]   Leslie SW, Sajjad H, Kumar S. Genital Warts.StatPearls. Treasure Island, FL: StatPearls Publishing 2022.https://www.ncbi.nlm.nih.gov/books/NBK441884/ Updated 2022 Nov 28

[14]   Irisawa R, Tsuboi R, Saito M, Harada K. Treatment of intra-anal warts with imiquimod 5% cream: A single-center prospective open study. J Dermatol 2021; 48(4): 476-80.

[http://dx.doi.org/10.1111/1346-8138.15759] [PMID: 33460189]

[15]   Kopera D, Kerl H. Visualization and treatment of subclinical actinic keratoses with topical imiquimod 5% cream: An observational study. BioMed Res Int 2014; 2014: 1-4.
[http://dx.doi.org/10.1155/2014/135916] [PMID: 24900953]

[16]   Rhodes J, Chen H, Hall SR, *et al.* Therapeutic potentiation of the immune system by costimulatory Schiff-base-forming drugs. Nature 1995; 377(6544): 71-5.
[http://dx.doi.org/10.1038/377071a0] [PMID: 7659167]

[17]   Manual   MSD.   Available   from: https://www.msdmanuals.com/professional/infectious-diseases/sexually-transmitted-infections-stis/human-papillomavirus-hpv-infection

[18]   Aggarwal S, Agarwal P, Singh AK. Human papilloma virus vaccines: A comprehensive narrative review. Cancer Treat Res Commun. 2023; 37: 100780. Epub 2023 Nov 21.
[http://dx.doi.org/10.1016/j.ctarc.2023.100780] [PMID: 38006748]

CHAPTER 18

Upton's Paste: An Extremely Potent Compound for Resistant Warts, Callouses and Corns

Mohammad Reza Namazi[1,*]

[1] *Shiraz University of Medical Sciences and Dr. Namazi Skin and Hair Clinic, Shiraz, Iran*

Though several options like cryotherapy and topical peeling agents, such as salicylic acid, are available for the treatment of verrucae, the treatment of resistant cases is challenging.

Upton's paste is composed of 60 g salicylic acid and 10 g trichloroacetic acid in glycerin (20g, or sufficient quantity to make a stiff paste). It is not mentioned in major textbooks but is remarkably effective against recalcitrant warts.

The Australian College of General Practitioners states that Upton's Paste is hugely potent and must be kept safely and only employed on the soles of the feet.

The patient's instructions are as follows [1]:

• File down the wart using a coarse emery board and throw away the board.

• Gently pinprick the wart to permit penetration of the paste into the wart.

• Paint clear nail polish on the normal skin around the wart.

• Cut a hole the same shape and size as the wart in a short strip of Elastoplast and apply to the area so that the wart is poking through the hole, but the surrounding skin must be protected from the paste.

• Apply the paste in small quantities.

• Cover with another strip of Elastoplast.

• Leave for 3 days.

* **Corresponding author Mohammad Reza Namazi:** Shiraz University of Medical Sciences and Dr. Namazi Skin and Hair Clinic, Shiraz, Iran; E-mail: rezanamazi12@yahoo.com

• Remove tape and wash, then with a cuticle stick or something similar, remove as much of the whitish necrotic material as possible without causing bleeding or pain.

• Leave overnight.

• Re-apply as above.

• After 3 days remove the Elastoplast in the morning and wash.

• Attend the same day as the Elastoplast has been removed for paring down the wart by the doctor.

An alternative, but being less strong, is 40%-60% salicylic acid in white soft paraffin. It is applied every day after showering and covered with waterproof tape. The wart is pared down once weekly with a sharp blade.

While I was a fellow in the dermatology department of Wake Forest University, USA, I noticed that the dermatologists used CPS: Cantharidine 1% + Podophylline 5% + SA 30% in an appropriate vehicle for common warts (applied by the physician).

REFERENCE

[1]   Available from: https://www.racgp.org.au / FSDEDEV / media / documents / Faculties / WA/ Instruction -on-the-use-of-Upton-s-paste.pdf

CHAPTER 19

Good Keratolytics for Non-irritated Thick Skin, *E.g.*, Lichen Simplex Chronicus and Keratosis Pilaris

Mohammad Reza Namazi[1,*]

[1] *Shiraz University of Medical Sciences and Dr. Namazi Skin and Hair Clinic, Shiraz, Iran*

Lichen simplex is a chronic, itchy skin condition characterized by well-demarcated plaques of thickened leathery skin. Keratosis pilaris, sometimes called "chicken skin" is a common skin condition presenting as patches of rough-feeling small papules on the skin.

20% propylene glycol + 4-6% lactic acid + 20% urea in eucerin is a good keratolytic and humectant for non-irritated thick skin, such as keratosis pilaris and acanthosis nigricans. Propylene glycol, lactic acid, and urea (if > 10%) all exert the keratolytic effect.

Keratosis pilaris shows a good response to 10% salicylic acid in vaseline as well. Salicylic acid is an anti-inflammatory agent that is keratolytic at concentrations of 3–6% and destructive at concentrations above 6%. Concentrations of 6–60% are used to remove corns and warts and in the treatment of psoriasis and other hyperkeratotic disorders [1]. Like urea, it is irritating at high concentrations in the acute inflammatory stage.

Also, Noreva Kerapil Cream, containing 14% ammonium lactate, is a good commercial product for these patients. Ammonium lactate contains lactic acid, an alpha hydroxy acid with keratolytic action. It is effective against ingrown hair and comedones as well.

For patients with very itchy, thick prurigo or nodular amyloidosis lesions, this formula works well, though you may need to use additional systemic therapy as well:

[*] **Corresponding author Mohammad Reza Namazi:** Shiraz University of Medical Sciences and Dr. Namazi Skin and Hair Clinic, Shiraz, Iran; E-mail: rezanamazi12@yahoo.com

0.5% menthol + 0.5% phenol + 0.5% camphor + 25% propylene glycol + 6% lactic acid + 20% urea q.s. eucerin (q.s.: Quantum satis, a Latin term meaning the amount which is enough; in this formulation, the rest of the mixture (47.4%) is composed of eucerin. If the concentration of eucerin is over 50%, we can use "in" instead of q.s.). The first three ingredients exert additive anti-pruritus effects, while the last three agents exert additive keratolytic and humectant effects. Urea has an anti-itch effect as well.

REFERENCE

[1]   Furman BL. Salicylic acid. Reference Module in Biomedical Sciences. Elsevier 2018.
        [http://dx.doi.org/10.1016/B978-0-12-801238-3.97758-4]

CHAPTER 20

Anti-histamines Pearls

Mohammad Reza Namazi[1,*]

[1] *Shiraz University of Medical Sciences and Dr. Namazi Skin and Hair Clinic, Shiraz, Iran*

Anti-histamines are prescribed to decrease the symptoms of type 1 allergic diseases (such as allergic rhinitis) and other conditions mediated by histamine, such as urticaria. Provided are some pearls regarding anti-histamines:

-Cetirizine and loratadine alleviate itching in atopic dermatitis [1]. They are in category B for use in pregnancy [1]. Chlorpheniramine is also considered safe in pregnancy, especially in the first two trimesters. A very small risk of neonatal seizure and respiratory depression is possible if chlorpheniramine is given shortly before birth [2].

- Breastfed infants whose mothers ingested first-generation anti-histamines may experience irritability, drowsiness or respiratory depression [1].

Loratadine/desloratadine and fexofenadine are excreted very minimally in breast milk, so these are the Anti-histamines of choice for breastfeeding mothers [3].

-While it is generally supposed that cetirizine does not cause sedation, in reality, many patients complain of its sedative side effect [4]. Consider loratadine or fexofenadine whenever sedation is not desirable.

- The use of anti-histamines, including fexofenadine and cetirizine, is associated with obesity. No information is available on the relative potency of anti-histamines regarding their effect on weight gain [5].

-Fexofenadine does not need dose adjustment in hepatic insufficiency [3].

-Levocetirizine and desloratadine have no drug interactions [5].

-Though doxepine can exert anti-depressant effects in addition to antihistamine effects, given its potent sedative and anti-cholinergic effects [6], it cannot be well tolerated by most patients, espescially the elderly. Benign prostatic hyperplasia,

[*] **Corresponding author Mohammad Reza Namazi:** Shiraz University of Medical Sciences and Dr. Namazi Skin and Hair Clinic, Shiraz, Iran; E-mail: rezanamazi12@yahoo.com

memory problems, heart rhythm disorders and constipation can worsen with anticholinergics. Precipitation of angle closure glaucoma and dry mouth are other side effects. Usually, managing the itch and the psychiatric problem with two, more tolerable medications is more tolerable by patients.

-Mirtazapine is a tetracyclic anti-depressant with potent anti-histamines properties. It also acts *via* central mechanisms to alleviate pruritus. Mirtazapine has a wide therapeutic index and virtually no anticholinergic effect. Mirtazapine may be an alternative therapy for pruritus that is refractory to first-line therapies or in depressed patients. It is started at 15 mg/night and increased every 1-2 weeks, if required, to the maximum dose of 45 mg/night. Maximum antidepressant effects of therapy may not be evident until ≥4 weeks. The main side effects of mirtazapine are heavy sedation, weight gain and hypercholesterolemia. Physicians should counsel patients to report worsening of depression or suicidal ideations. Mirtazapine cannot be prescribed if the patient has used an MAO inhibitor, such as linezolid, in the past 14 days because of the risk of serotonin syndrome [7, 8].

REFERENCES

[1]   Motala C. H1 anti-histamines in allergic disease. Curr Allergy Clin Immunol 2009; 22(2): 71-4.

[2]   Wakelin SH. Handbook of Systemic Drug Treatment in Dermatology. London: Manson Publishing Ltd 2002; pp. 70-218.
[http://dx.doi.org/10.1201/b16367]

[3]   Dávila I, del Cuvillo A, Mullol J, *et al.* Use of second generation H1 anti-histamines in special situations. J Investig Allergol Clin Immunol 2013; 23 (Suppl. 1): 1-16.
[PMID: 24672890]

[4]   Falliers CJ, Brandon ML, Buchman E, *et al.* Double-blind comparison of cetirizine and placebo in the treatment of seasonal rhinitis. Ann Allergy 1991; 66(3): 257-62.
[PMID: 1672494]

[5]   Ratliff JC, Barber JA, Palmese LB, Reutenauer EL, Tek C. Association of prescription H1 antihistamine use with obesity: Results from the national health and nutrition examination survey. Obesity 2010; 18(12): 2398-400.
[http://dx.doi.org/10.1038/oby.2010.176] [PMID: 20706200]

[6]   Namazi MR. Prescribing cyclic anti-depressants for vitiligo patients: Which agents are superior, which are not? Psychother Psychosom 2003; 72(6): 361-2.
[http://dx.doi.org/10.1159/000073036] [PMID: 14526142]

[7]   Khanna R, Boozalis E, Belzberg M, Zampella JG, Kwatra SG. Mirtazapine for the treatment of chronic pruritus. Medicines 2019; 6(3): 73.
[http://dx.doi.org/10.3390/medicines6030073] [PMID: 31284577]

[8]   Drugs.com website. Mitrazapine. 2023. Available from: https://www.drugs.com/monograph/mirtazapine.html (Accessesd: 1/4/2023).

CHAPTER 21

Acne Management: Pearls

Mohammad Reza Namazi[1,*]

[1] *Shiraz University of Medical Sciences and Dr. Namazi Skin and Hair Clinic, Shiraz, Iran*

Acne is one of the most common conditions seen by dermatologists. Some useful tips on the management of acne are presented here:

-In papular acne patients, azithromycin can be added to isotretinoin to keep the dosage of isotretinoin lower (in severe patients or cases intolerant to isotretinoin-induced xerosis). For example, by prescribing the two agents on alternate days, control on acne can be achieved with less xerotic effect from isotretinoin.

Note that if the acne has comedonal components, oral antibiotics cannot be helpful in resolving the comedones and the only effective oral agent is isotretinoin.

In females, spironolactone or flutamide can be added to isotretinoin to keep the dose of isotretinoin lower.

-The combination of oral azithromycin and topical benzoylperoxide prevents the formation of *P.acnes* resistant to azithromycin [1].

-Make sure to advise acne patients to use oil-free sunscreens and non-comedogenic moisturizers in case they experience isotretinoin-induced xerosis, otherwise, they may use products made for dry skin, which can exacerbate the acne.

-Do not prescribe a face wash or soap suitable for oily skin if you have prescribed isotretinoin, as the patient's face becomes very dry and irritated. In my experience, Kapus Doctor's soap and Kapus Protective soap are good choices for acne patients on isotretinoin, as these soaps do not dry the skin. Instead, you may prescribe formulations for normal skin but not for oily or dry skin. A formulation suitable for dry skin may cause the skin to become oily.

---

* **Corresponding author Mohammad Reza Namazi:** Shiraz University of Medical Sciences and Dr. Namazi Skin and Hair Clinic, Shiraz, Iran; E-mail: rezanamazi12@yahoo.com

-Alcohol based topicals, such as benzoyl peroxide gel, may not be tolerable by the patients on isotretinoin as it dries the skin.

-When the patient's acne resolves, I usually decrease the dose of isotretinoin, *e.g.*, to 2-3 capsules per week, and if there is no recurrence in 2-3 months, I discontinue it and only re-start upon recurrence. I do not believe that giving a fixed total dose of isotretinoin, as mentioned in some publications, can prevent the recurrence of acne. No scientific explanation is provided for this claim, and my own experience also does not support it.

-Some female patients with resistant acne have normal menses and no hirsutism or hair loss but have high prolactin levels. Consider checking hormone levels in resistant or severe acne patients even if the menses are normal and there is no lactorrhea.

-In the author's experience, Uriage Hyseac 50+ fluid sunscreen is suitable for acne patients, as it contains some ingredients that provide a lasting mattifying effect by decreasing seborrhea while reducing dehydration.

- Commercial topical products effective against both papular and comedonal acne are not available in all regions. For this clinical scenario, the following topicals can be prescribed:

• 1% clindamycin + 10% propylen glycol + 2-3% salicylic acid in Alcohol 70°

• 2-4% erythromycin + 10% propylen glycol + 2-3% salicylic acid in Alcohol 70°

-Multiple studies and meta-analyses have now confirmed that for patients taking isotretinoin, if baseline blood and peak dose blood (at 8 weeks) are normal, no further testing is needed. However, if 8-week blood is abnormal, periodic testing is required [2].

REFERENCES

[1]   Stein Gold L, Baldwin H, Kircik LH, *et al.* Efficacy and safety of a fixed-dose clindamycin phosphate 1.2%, benzoyl peroxide 3.1%, and adapalene 0.15% gel for moderate-to-severe acne: a randomized phase II study of the first triple-combination drug. Am J Clin Dermatol 2022; 23(1): 93-104.
[http://dx.doi.org/10.1007/s40257-021-00650-3] [PMID: 34674160]

[2]   Jiyad Z, Flohr C. Handbook of Skin Disease Management. 1st ed. India: John Wiley & Sons Ltd. 2023; p. 189.
[http://dx.doi.org/10.1002/9781119829072]

CHAPTER 22

Which Topicals are Appropriate for Acne Patients with Dry Skin?

Mohammad Reza Namazi[1,*]

[1] *Shiraz University of Medical Sciences and Dr. Namazi Skin and Hair Clinic, Shiraz, Iran*

There are many acne patients who, surprisingly, have xerotic skin. Prescribing topical clindamycin and erythromycin solutions, which have an alcoholic base, or benzoyl peroxide, can irritate their skin. Below, some novel compounds are presented. Note that topical antibiotics are effective against papular acne and not against comedonal acne [1].

If the skin is very dry, prescribe the following compounds:

• 1% clindamycin powder in an oil-free moisturizer (*e.g.*, Sebium Hydra, made by Bioderma).

• 4% erythromycin powder in an oil-free moisturizer (*e.g.*, Sebium Hydra). 25% benzoyl peroxide 10% solution (in fact, 2.5% benzoyl peroxide) can be added to the formula to have a stronger anti-acne effect while preventing the resistance of P. acne to erythromycin: 4% erythromycin powder + 25% benzoyl peroxide 10 solution in Sebium Hydra.

A gel base can be used if the skin is not very dry:

2-4% Erythromycin powder +/- 25% benzoylperoxide 10 solution [= 2.5% benzoylperoxide] in gel base. Expert pharmacists can make a non-greasy gel using carboxymethyl cellulose. KY jelly is not a good base as it transforms into a sticky film after application, which is not liked by patients.

For comedonal acne patients intolerant to tretinoin and adapalen, Sebium Global, made by Bioderma, can be considered. It contains AHA esters, zinc gluconate, *etc*. and is effective against comedones. It is mattifying, *i.e.*, decreases facial shininess, and moisturising, and is not irritating.

* **Corresponding author Mohammad Reza Namazi:** Shiraz University of Medical Sciences and Dr. Namazi Skin and Hair Clinic, Shiraz, Iran; E-mail: rezanamazi12@yahoo.com

To decrease the chance of irritation by adapalene or tretinoin, advise patients to apply the medication in a small amount as a thin smear at least two hours after washing the face and to avoid massaging it onto the skin. Neither of the agents is photosensitive. Adapalene is less irritating than tretinoin. The patients can apply them less frequently (*e.g.*, every other night) in case they experience skin irritation.

If you need to prescribe isotretinoin for an acne patient with dry skin, you have to prescribe a non-comedogenic emollient (like Sebium Hydra) along with it to prevent excessive facial dryness, which can undermine the patient's adherence.

Acne patients with dry skin frequently use greasy moisturizers, even petrolatum, which exacerbates their acne. It is important to advise them to use oil-free moisturizers even if they have dry skin.

In the author's experience, topical isotretinoin is not very effective against acne.

REFERENCE

[1]   Huang CY, Chang IJ, Bolick N, *et al.* Comparative efficacy of pharmacological treatments for acne vulgaris: A network meta-analysis of 221 randomized controlled trials. Ann Fam Med 2023; 21(4): 358-69.
[http://dx.doi.org/10.1370/afm.2995] [PMID: 37487721]

CHAPTER 23

Melasma Pearls

Mohammad Reza Namazi[1,*]

[1] *Shiraz University of Medical Sciences and Dr. Namazi Skin and Hair Clinic, Shiraz, Iran*

Melasma is a common skin disorder. The most effective formulation against melasma is a combination of hydroquinone, tretinoin, and moderate-potency topical steroids. Herein, some effective formulations are discussed:

-2% Hydroquinone (HQ) powder + 10% adapalene cream + 10% mometasone cream + 3% vit C powder in cold cream (Adapalene cream = Adapalene cream 0.1%; Mometasone cream = Mometasone cream 0.1%).

A gel base made by some expert pharmacists may be used instead of cold cream for oily skin.

In this formulation, vitamin C prevents oxidation of HQ. It is important that the pharmacist uses vitamin C powder and not crushed vitamin C tablets, as the tablets have some excipients which can cause contact dermatitis. For making this compound, pharmacists use adapalene cream 0.1%, therefore, the concentration of adapalene is 0.01% in the compound. Tretinoin is not used as it is more irritating than adapalene. Also, pharmacists use mometasone cream 0.1%, so the concentration of mometasone is 0.01% in the compound. Mometasone has the least atrophogenic potential than other potent topical steroids.

If 4% HQ is used, which is significantly more irritating than 2% HQ, the formulation can be changed to 4% HQ + 10% adapalene cream + 5% vit C powder in mometasone cream, to curb irritation more strongly by a higher concentration of mometasone, or preferably to 4% HQ powder + 4% salicylic acid + 4% nicotinamide powder + 30% eucerin + 5% vit C powder in mometasone cream. 5% HQ can be used in very resistant cases. In the latter formulation, 4% salicylic acid is used instead of adapalene, which can irritate the skin. Salicylic acid increases the penetration of other agents, including HQ, and also exerts anti-inflammatory effects. Nicotinamide has both skin-lightening and anti-inflamma-

[*] **Corresponding author Mohammad Reza Namazi:** Shiraz University of Medical Sciences and Dr. Namazi Skin and Hair Clinic, Shiraz, Iran; E-mail: rezanamazi12@yahoo.com

tory effects. Eucerin is a good base for both lipid and water-soluble ingredients and helps in keeping the ingredients together.

The HQ-containing compounds should be applied at night in a very small amount and NOT massaged on the skin. Massage increases the likelihood of irritation. The patient should not wash his/her face for at least 2 hours prior to the application to prevent irritation. Application of a moisturizer prior to HQ can mitigate its irritation. After application, the patient should turn off bright lights, but dim lights are acceptable. HQ-containing formulations frequently cause phototoxicity in summer in sunny climates, especially in people engaging in outdoor activities and are usually not tolerated in these situations.

After the resolution of melasma, which usually takes 2-3 months or so, discontinuing skin-lightening agents usually causes recurrence. Maintenance application of the skin-lightening agents two nights per week can prevent a recurrence.

-Another formulation:

2% HQ + 10% adapalene cream + 10% mometasone cream + 2% nicotinamide powder + 3% vit C powder in cold cream.

For resistant melasma, it is possible to keep the concentration of HQ to 2% and add 15-20% azelaic acid. Azelaic acid 20% is equal to HQ 2% in efficacy but is less irritating:

2% HQ + 20% azelaic acid powder + 4% salicylic acid + 4% nicotinamide + 30% eucerin + 3% vit C powder in mometasone cream.

Please note that though azelaic acid is considered non-irritating, it sometimes causes irritation on sensitive skin. However, it is definitely much less irritating than hydroquinone. Nicotinamide exerts both skin-lightening and anti-inflammatory effects.

Oral tranexamic acid, 500 mg BD for 12 weeks, can be considered for the treatment of melasma unresponsive to hydroquinone. History of venous or arterial thrombosis, severe renal impairment, and convulsion are contraindications to its use. Despite a theoretical risk of thromboembolism, studies have shown that tranexamic acid does not increase the thromboembolic risk [1]; however, an overcautious clinician can consider co-prescribing aspirin for safeguarding against thrombosis.

Regarding the use of sunscreen in melasma patients, it is suggested that not only ultraviolet (UV) but also visible light (VL) is involved in the pathogenesis of melasma.UV-VL sunscreens enhance the depigmenting efficacy of hydroquinone compared with UV-only sunscreens. Therefore, the use of tinted sunscreens is recommended for these patients [2].

Sunscreen SPFs are labeled by testing at an application density of 2 mg/cm^2, however, consumer application densities range from 0.5 to 1 mg/cm^2. Therefore, sunscreens with SPF 70 and above, in contrast to sunscreens with lower SPF values, add additional clinical benefit by delivering an actual SPF that meets the minimum SPF levels recommended for photodamage prevention [3]. This is also of importance in the prevention of hydroquinone-induced phototoxicity.

Sunsense Sport Milk is a four-hour water-resistant SPF 50+ roll-on sunscreen made in Australia, best suited to those engaging in outdoor activities. It is non-greasy and very suitable for men and those with oily skin. As it can be applied every four hours, in contrast to two hours, which is usual for sunscreens, it can resolve the problem of patients' inadequate application of sunscreens, which contributes to the relapse of melasma.

REFERENCES

[1]   Bala HR, Lee S, Wong C, Pandya AG, Rodrigues M. Oral tranexamic acid for the treatment of melasma: A review. Dermatol Surg 2018; 44(6): 814-25.
        [http://dx.doi.org/10.1097/DSS.0000000000001518] [PMID: 29677015]

[2]   Castanedo-Cazares JP, Hernandez-Blanco D, Carlos-Ortega B, Fuentes-Ahumada C, Torres-Álvarez B. Near-visible light and UV photoprotection in the treatment of melasma: A double-blind randomized trial. Photodermatol Photoimmunol Photomed 2014; 30(1): 35-42.
        [http://dx.doi.org/10.1111/phpp.12086] [PMID: 24313385]

[3]   Ou-Yang H, Stanfield J, Cole C, Appa Y, Rigel D. High-SPF sunscreens (SPF ≥ 70) may provide ultraviolet protection above minimal recommended levels by adequately compensating for lower sunscreen user application amounts. J Am Acad Dermatol 2012; 67(6): 1220-7.
        [http://dx.doi.org/10.1016/j.jaad.2012.02.029] [PMID: 22463921]

CHAPTER 24

How to Make a Strong Anti-Acne and Anti-Pigment Agent?

Mohammad Reza Namazi[1,*]

[1] *Shiraz University of Medical Sciences and Dr. Namazi Skin and Hair Clinic, Shiraz, Iran*

Managing a patient with both acne and melasma is a challenge. Provided are some helpful tips for this clinical situation:

-The following compound can be prescribed to improve both acne and melasma/acne-induced hyperpigmentation:

Azelaic acid 20% + nicotinamide 2-4% in gel base. Both the agents are effective against both the conditions. Also, it is possible to mix nicotinamide powder with commercial azelaic acid gels (2-4% nicotinamide in azelaic acid gel). Though azelaic acid is supposed to be anti-inflammatory [1], azelaic acid preparations sometimes irritate sensitive skin. The anti-inflammatory effect of nicotinamide prevents azelaic acid-induced irritation. Salicylic acid 2% can be added to further curb the irritation of azelaic acid and increase its penetration. Salicylic acid has a comedolytic effect as well.

Both azelaic acid and nicotinamide are in category B in pregnancy.

REFERENCES

[1] Burkhart CG, Katz KA. Other topical medications. In: Goldsmith LA, Katz SI, Gilchrest BA, Paller AS, Leffell AJ, Wolf K, Eds. Other topical medications In: Fitzpatrick's Dermatology in General Medicine. 8th ed. USA: McGraw-Hill 2012; pp. 2697-707.

* **Corresponding author Mohammad Reza Namazi:** Shiraz University of Medical Sciences and Dr. Namazi Skin and Hair Clinic, Shiraz, Iran; E-mail: rezanamazi12@yahoo.com

CHAPTER 25

How to Treat Peri-Orbital Hypermelanosis and Melasma in Sensitive Skin?

Mohammad Reza Namazi[1,*]

[1] *Shiraz University of Medical Sciences and Dr. Namazi Skin and Hair Clinic, Shiraz, Iran*

Hyperpigmentation of sensitive eyelids is a relatively challenging condition to treat, as hydroquinone-containing creams, which are very effective anti-pigment agents, can be irritating on delicate skin. Some other non-irritating topicals, such as creams containing glabridin, a licorice extract, can also be helpful. An example is Trio-A, made by Noreva. Licorice is not only a tyrosinase inhibitor but also an anti-inflammatory agent [1]. Photoderm Spot is an antisolar containing licorice that can be applied on the eyelids. The following compound can exert a more potent skin-lightening effect on sensitive skin:

-2-4% nicotinamide in Trio-A cream $\neq$ 30 ml (Trio-A comes in 30 ml tubes)

Pharmaceris W day cream is a 50+ anti-solar containing vitamin C and nicotinamide. Nicotinamide is an anti-inflammatory and skin-lightening agent [2]. Pharmaceris W night cream is a skin-lightening cream containing vitamin C and nicotinamide, which can be used for sensitive skin. However, these non-irritating creams are usually not as potent as hydroquinone-containing creams.

Another good option is mesotherapy with a tranexamic acid-vitamin C mixture every other week; both agents are tyrosinase inhibitors. Mesotherapy can be combined with topicals.

REFERENCES

[1]   Yokota T, Nishio H, Kubota Y, Mizoguchi M. The inhibitory effect of glabridin from licorice extracts on melanogenesis and inflammation. Pigment Cell Res 1998; 11(6): 355-61.
[http://dx.doi.org/10.1111/j.1600-0749.1998.tb00494.x] [PMID: 9870547]

[2]   Namazi MR. Nicotinamide in dermatology: A capsule summary. Int J Dermatol 2007; 46(12): 1229-31.
[http://dx.doi.org/10.1111/j.1365-4632.2007.03519.x] [PMID: 18173513]

---

[*] **Corresponding author Mohammad Reza Namazi:** Shiraz University of Medical Sciences and Dr. Namazi Skin and Hair Clinic, Shiraz, Iran; E-mail: rezanamazi12@yahoo.com

CHAPTER 26

Doxycycline or Azithromycin for Perifollicular Elastolysis?

Mohammad Reza Namazi[1,*]

[1] *Shiraz University of Medical Sciences and Dr. Namazi Skin and Hair Clinic, Shiraz, Iran*

Papular acne scars consist of small, asymptomatic, hypopigmented, follicular papules on the upper part of the trunk. Biopsy shows circumscribed, peri- or para-follicular lesions in which both elastic and collagen fibers are decreased.

The perifollicular papular scars are considered a scarring process secondary to acne vulgaris. They appear closely related to or identical with changes previously termed, *i.e.*, perifollicular elastolysis, post-acne anetoderma-like scars, and papular elastorrhexis [1].

Pathogenesis of dermal elastolysis, including perifollicular elastolysis, remains obscure. Elastic fiber degradation occurs secondary either to an increased synthesis of elastases or to an imbalance between activated matrix metalloproteinases (MMPs) and their natural inhibitors [2]. Doxycycline is an inhibitor of MMPs [3], and therefore, it is favored over azithromycin for treating acne complicated by perifollicular elastolysis. More effective treatment with isotretinoin for the prevention of this condition is prudent. Doxycycline may prove to be effective in other conditions associated with decreased elastic fibers, such as atrophia maculosa varioliformis cutis.

REFERENCES

[1]   Wilson BB, Dent CH, Cooper PH. Papular acne scars. A common cutaneous finding. Arch Dermatol 1990; 126(6): 797-800.
[http://dx.doi.org/10.1001/archderm.1990.01670300097016] [PMID: 2140672]

[2]   Zheng Y, Su X, Chen Z, Han L. Perifollicular elastolysis caused by repeatedly shaving armpit hairs. J Cosmet Dermatol 2021; 20(8): 2673-4.
[http://dx.doi.org/10.1111/jocd.13901] [PMID: 33355989]

[3]   AAssar OS, Fujiwara NH, Marx WF, Matsumoto AH, Kallmes DF. Aneurysm growth, elastinolysis, and attempted doxycycline inhibition of elastase-induced aneurysms in rabbits. J Vasc Interv Radiol 2003; 14(11): 1427-32.
[http://dx.doi.org/10.1097/01.RVI.0000096772.74047.13] [PMID: 14605108]

[*] **Corresponding author Mohammad Reza Namazi:** Shiraz University of Medical Sciences and Dr. Namazi Skin and Hair Clinic, Shiraz, Iran; E-mail: rezanamazi12@yahoo.com

CHAPTER 27

Excessive Skin Oiliness: Tips

Mohammad Reza Namazi[1,*]

¹ Shiraz University of Medical Sciences and Dr. Namazi Skin and Hair Clinic, Shiraz, Iran

Excessively oily skin, called seborrhea, is due to overactive sebaceous glands.

Most people with seborrhoea are otherwise healthy, however, it may be a sign of Parkinson's disease, acromegaly, prolactinoma, hyperthyroidism, or hyperandrogenism in women [1].

How to know whether a patient has dry, oily, or normal skin? It is simple: ask them whether they have dry or oily skin. They will answer "dry", "oily", or "I don't know". If they answer "I don't know", they have normal skin.

No standard topical agent is mentioned in major textbooks for managing facial oiliness. However, some commercial topical agents are helpful. An example is Esthederm Pure System, which decreases facial greasiness and shininess and can also reduce pore size to some extent. Wheat germ soap is also very effective in decreasing facial oiliness.

Ketoconazole shampoo reduces scalp oiliness due to its anti-androgenic effect. It is also effective against androgenic alopecia [2]. Most patients using ketoconazole shampoo for dandruff complain of its drying effect.

If severe and especially generalized, oral isotretinoin can be very helpful for skin oiliness. In women, anti-androgens are effective.

Botulinum toxin injection reduces sebum secretion, suggesting that nerve-derived substances modulate sebocyte functions [1].

Sebocytes mainly have 5-alpha-reductase type 1, therefore, finasteride, a blocker of the type 2 enzyme, cannot reduce seborrhea [1].

* **Corresponding author Mohammad Reza Namazi:** Shiraz University of Medical Sciences and Dr. Namazi Skin and Hair Clinic, Shiraz, Iran; E-mail: rezanamazi12@yahoo.com

REFERENCES

[1]   Clayton RW, Langan EA, Ansell DM, *et al.* Neuroendocrinology and neurobiology of sebaceous glands. Biol Rev Camb Philos Soc 2020; 95(3): 592-624.
[http://dx.doi.org/10.1111/brv.12579] [PMID: 31970855]

[2]   Fields JR, Vonu PM, Monir RL, Schoch JJ. Topical ketoconazole for the treatment of androgenetic alopecia: A systematic review. Dermatol Ther 2020; 33(1)e13202
[http://dx.doi.org/10.1111/dth.13202] [PMID: 31858672]

CHAPTER 28

Enlarged Pores

Mohammad Reza Namazi[1,*]

[1] *Shiraz University of Medical Sciences and Dr. Namazi Skin and Hair Clinic, Shiraz, Iran*

Enlarged pores are a very common aesthetic complaint. Facial pores are openings to the ducts of the sebaceous glands.

Factors that may lead to enlarged pores include seborrhea (see the previous section), use of comedogenic products, inflammatory acne, loss of skin elasticity with age, sun damage, and big hair follicle size [1].

Treatments that focus on preventing and shrinking large pores are not very effective, such as chemical peels, topical retinoids, etc. The author did not find Sebium Pore Refiner, made by Bioderma, to be very effective.

Oral treatments that are used for acne might help, such as combined oral contraceptives, spironolactone, and isotretinoin.

Physical treatments targeting the sebaceous glands may help, such as radiofrequency microneedling.

REFERENCE

[1]   Dermnet. Enlarged pores. Available from: https://dermnetnz.org/topics/enlarged-pores (Accessed 9/28/2022).

[*] **Corresponding author Mohammad Reza Namazi:** Shiraz University of Medical Sciences and Dr. Namazi Skin and Hair Clinic, Shiraz, Iran; E-mail: rezanamazi12@yahoo.com

CHAPTER 29

Facial Erythema

Mohammad Reza Namazi[1,*]

[1] Shiraz University of Medical Sciences and Dr. Namazi Skin and Hair Clinic, Shiraz, Iran

Facial erythema may be caused by many disorders, such as phototoxic and photoallergic reactions, lupus erythematosus, dermatomyositis, diabetes, rosacea, polymorphous light eruption, contact dermatitis, topical steroid withdrawal, *etc* [1].

Sometimes, no specific etiologic cause can be identified for facial erythema.

Brimonidine and oxymetazoline gels, neuromodulators (injecting BOTOX, 1 U every 1 cm), and lasers (PDL, etc) are used for the treatment of facial erythema [1].

A patient with erythematotelangiectatic rosacea unresponsive to doxycycline, clonidine, and pimecrolimus cream 1% responded dramatically to carvedilol, 6.25 mg twice a day for the first week, followed by 3 times a day thereafter. Carvedilol is approved for treating mild to moderate congestive heart failure and is well tolerated even in the elderly, with lower rates of hypotension (3.3%) and bradycardia (1.7%) compared to propranolol. However, it is prudent to monitor patients for side effects. Carvedilol has more potent antioxidant properties compared with other beta-blockers [2].

Sensibio Forte is a cream made by Bioderma that quickly resolves skin inflammation and augments the tolerance threshold of the skin. Its soothing ingredients, including allantoin and enoxolone, quickly resolve redness. A patented complex makes the skin less reactive, and some moisturising agents resolve skin dehydration that often accompanies irritation. Sensibio Forte can also be used for erythema seen after shaving, hair removal, peeling, post-laser, solar erythema, *etc* [3].

* **Corresponding author Mohammad Reza Namazi:** Shiraz University of Medical Sciences and Dr. Namazi Skin and Hair Clinic, Shiraz, Iran; E-mail: rezanamazi12@yahoo.com

Photoderm AR is a 50+ sunscreen that resolves skin erythema. It is a non-sticky, non-greasy, non-comedogenic, unfragranced, and water-resistant cream with very good cutaneous and ocular tolerance [4].

REFERENCES

[1]   Loyal J, Carr E, Almukhtar R, Goldman MP. Updates and best practices in the management of facial erythema. Clin Cosmet Investig Dermatol 2021; 14: 601-14.
        [http://dx.doi.org/10.2147/CCID.S267203] [PMID: 34135612]

[2]   Hsu CC, Lee JY. Carvedilol for the treatment of refractory facial flushing and persistent erythema of rosacea. Arch Dermatol 2011; 147(11): 1258-60.
        [http://dx.doi.org/10.1001/archdermatol.2011.204] [PMID: 21768447]

[3]   Bioderma Website. Available from: https://www.bioderma.ae/our-products/sensibio/forte (Accessed 9/23/2022).

[4]   Bioderma Website. Available from: https://www.bioderma.co.uk/our-products/photoderm/ar-spf50 (Accessed 9/23/022).

CHAPTER 30

What is an Excellent Anti-Redness Emollient for Ichthyosiform Erythroderma?

Mohammad Reza Namazi[1,*]

[1] *Shiraz University of Medical Sciences and Dr. Namazi Skin and Hair Clinic, Shiraz, Iran*

Managing both erythema and excessive xerosis seen in ichthyosiform erythroderma is not easy. Below, some effective compound formulations are discussed:

-3% urea + 2% lactic acid + 2% nicotinamide + 5% glycerin in eucerin is very effective in the author's experience. Nicotinamide exerts remarkable anti-inflammatory effects and improves the skin barrier function [1]. It is usually used at 2-4% concentrations in cosmeceuticals. Higher concentrations can be irritating. It is advisable to keep its concentration to 2% for very irritated skin. 10% dexpanthenol cream 5% can be added to the formula. 0.5% menthol can be added if the patient is suffering from severe itch.

-For lamellar ichthyosis, 15% urea + 15-20% propylene glycol + 2-5% lactic acid in eucerin is a good keratolytic moisturizer. The combination of urea, lactic acid and propylene glycol causes an additive keratolytic effect without causing irritation. For very irritated skin, lower concentrations of propylene glycol (10-15%) and lactic acid (2%) can be used.

• Propylene glycol is a humectant, occlusive, and keratolytic agent that increases the penetration of medications and is used in most commercial products. A combination of 20% propylene glycol and 5% lactic acid in a semiocclusive cream base is used as a highly effective, well-tolerated keratolytic in lamellar ichthyosis [2]. Higher propylene glycol concentrations can be irritating to damaged skin.

• The keratolytic effect of urea starts at 10% concentration. Urea is a humectant that has a good water-binding capacity and facilitates epidermal barrier regeneration. Urea has keratolytic and antimicrobial effects. It should be avoided

[*] **Corresponding author Mohammad Reza Namazi:** Shiraz University of Medical Sciences and Dr. Namazi Skin and Hair Clinic, Shiraz, Iran; E-mail: rezanamazi12@yahoo.com

in newborns because of irritation and the risk of increased blood levels [3]. It should be used at a 3% concentration in children.

• Glycerin is a humectant that increases the degradation of desmosomes and is especially helpful in patients with ichthyosis [4].

-Traupe and Burgdorf [3] believed that regular bathing is helpful for ichthyosis patients as scales are loosened. They pointed out that adding several handfuls of sodium bicarbonate ($NaHCO_3$, baking soda) to a tub of water is very effective in denaturing keratin and removing the scales.

REFERENCES

[1]   Namazi MR. Nicotinamide: A potential addition to the anti-psoriatic weaponry. FASEB J 2003; 17(11): 1377-9.
        [http://dx.doi.org/10.1096/fj.03-0002hyp] [PMID: 12890690]

[2]   Burkhart CG, Katz KA. Other topical medications. In: Goldsmith LA, Katz SI, Gilchrest BA, Paller AS, Leffell AJ, Wolf K, Eds. Other topical medications In: Fitzpatrick's Dermatology in General Medicine. 8th ed. USA: McGraw-Hill 2012; pp. 2697-707.

[3]   Traupe H, Burgdorf WHC. Treatment of ichthyosis–There is always something you can do! In Memoriam: Wolfgang Küster. J Am Acad Dermatol 2007; 57(3): 542-7.
        [http://dx.doi.org/10.1016/j.jaad.2007.03.039]

[4]   Metz M, Staubach P. Itch management: Topical agents. Curr Probl Dermatol 2016; 50: 40-5.
        [http://dx.doi.org/10.1159/000446040] [PMID: 27578070]

CHAPTER 31

Pemphigus Pearls

Mohammad Reza Namazi[1,*]

[1] *Shiraz University of Medical Sciences and Dr. Namazi Skin and Hair Clinic, Shiraz, Iran*

Pemphigus is a potentially fatal blistering disease that is more common in Eastern people like Iranians. Below, some pearls on the management of this serious disease are given:

- Usually, oral candidiasis in pemphigus patients is resistant to fluconazole; using itraconazole is therefore recommended.

-A common mis-management is starting low-dose prednisolone in pemphigus patients having only oral disease, especially if severe. Oral pemphigus is usually as stubborn as the cutaneous-oral type, at least in Caucasians. Though some textbooks mention topical steroids to be effective against pemphigus vulgaris, this author has not found them particularly effective.

-In Eastern people, pemphigus and bullous pemphigoid are much stubborner than in Western people, and it is not advised to use the low steroid doses mentioned in Western textbooks.

-Though some *in vitro* studies have shown the pivotal role of urokinase-type plasminogen activator (uPA) in the pathogenesis of pemphigus vulgaris [1], I have not found tranexamic acid, an inhibitor of uPA, to be effective in this disease. This is not surprising given that not infrequently the results of *in vitro*, *in vivo* and even animal studies are not endorsed by clinical studies/experience.

-Some researchers believe that acantholysis depends not only on anti-desmoglein antibodies (Abs) but also on other antibodies produced against keratinocyte membrane antigens (*e.g.*, anti-acetylcholine (ACH) receptor antibodies). They mention that in the initial phase of pemphigus, anti-Ach receptor antibodies prevent Ach signaling necessary for intercellular adhesion as well as cell shape. *In vitro* studies demonstrate that large doses of Ach can quickly reverse acantholysis. Also, *in vivo* studies on a neonatal mice model of pemphigus have shown that

[*] **Corresponding author Mohammad Reza Namazi:** Shiraz University of Medical Sciences and Dr. Namazi Skin and Hair Clinic, Shiraz, Iran; E-mail: rezanamazi12@yahoo.com

cholinergic agonists decrease the lesions [2]. I have theorized that gargling with cholinergic ocular drops can help in the treatment of oral pemphigus vulgaris [3], however, my clinical experience in this regard has been futile. In my experience, anticholinergics, including physostigmine (Mestinon), do not provide any remarkable benefit in this disease. This is not surprising given that not infrequently *in vitro*, *in vivo* and even animal studies are not supported by clinical experience/studies.

-Pulse therapy rapidly controls severe pemphigus and dramatically decreases hospitalization time and is therefore highly encouraged [4] (See the chapter on Pulse Steroid Therapy). Oral doses are usually continued following pulse therapy [5].

Methylprednisolone, 2 mg/kg/day administered every 6-8 hours, can also be used to control severe diseases [5].

Gheisari *et al*. [4] used the following protocol for pulse therapy in pemphigus, though as mentioned in the chapter on Steroid Pulse therapy, non-intensive monitoring is acceptable for those without underlying medical conditions who do not have severe pemphigus:

Negative results for hepatitis B, hepatitis C, HIV, and T.B. tests, as well as normal EKG, are required for instigating pulse therapy.

Methylprednisolone (as sodium succinate) is administered at 20–30 mg kg/d (maximum dose of 1 g) for four consecutive days. It is dissolved in 200 ml of 5% dextrose and infused slowly over 2–3 hours. The patient's heart rate, respiratory rate, and blood pressure are checked every 15 min during the infusion and then every 6 hours after the completion of treatment for 24 hours. The infusion is discontinued if arrhythmia or hypertension occurs. Then, after cardiac consultation and correction of hemodynamic issues, the infusion is re-commenced at a much slower rate. Laboratory tests, including levels of blood sugar and potassium and EKG, are checked 6 hours after the termination of pulse therapy. Patients are examined on the following day after the completion of the course of pulse therapy. If new lesions cease to occur and Nikolsky's sign is negative, then oral prednisolone (0.5 mg/kg/day) and azathioprine (1-1.5 mg/kg/d) are started, and the patient is discharged after a few days. Recalcitrant patients receive another course of pulse therapy every month [The author of this chapter believes that additional courses can be given after one week to control re-calcitrant disease].

At the end of each course of pulse therapy, the dosage of maintenance oral prednisolone is decreased by 5 mg. Monthly pulse therapy courses are ceased if the patients are in complete remission (absence of new bullae and healing of the already present lesions by 80%). Usually, 1-6 sessions are needed to achieve remission. After the termination of the monthly pulse therapy, oral prednisolone is tapered as follows: the dosages higher than 20 mg/d are tapered by 5 mg per month. At 20 mg/d, the dosage is decreased by 2.5 mg per month to reach the dosage of 5 mg/d (in case of complete remission). At this time, the adjuvant drug is tapered. If any relapse is noted in the monthly visits, the adjuvant dose is increased, or further pulses are given until complete remission is achieved, and then tapering is resumed. To taper the adjuvant (after the patient's prednisolone is reached to 5 mg /d), the dose of the adjuvant drug is decreased monthly to half of the last dose for two months, and then the adjuvant is discontinued. Once the patient is receiving oral prednisolone at just 5 mg/d without adjuvant (about 1 year since starting treatment), treatment is ceased based on the negative direct immunofluorescence or the normal titer of serum antibodies.

- In the author's experience, azathioprine is more effective than mycophenolate as an adjuvant, as Chams-Davatch *et al.* have also noticed [6].

-Rituximab is a monoclonal antibody against CD20 that destructs autoreactive B cells. Its effect lasts six to nine months.

- Rituximab is indicated for patients who do not respond sufficiently to conventional medications or in whom systemic steroids and/or other immunosuppressives are contraindicated or cause severe side effects. It is also indicated in patients who relapse following treatment with conventional treatment. Some experts used rituximab as a first-line agent, especially in severe pemphigus [7].

-Patients with chronic oral pemphigus cannot eat sour food and, therefore, may be vitamin C deficient, which can negatively affect the healing of their lesions.

REFERENCES

[1]   Feliciani C, Toto P, Wang B, Sauder DN, Amerio P, Tulli A. Urokinase plasminogen activator mRNA is induced by IL-1α and TNF-α in *in vitro* acantholysis. Exp Dermatol 2003; 12(4): 466-71.
[http://dx.doi.org/10.1034/j.1600-0625.2002.120415.x] [PMID: 12930304]

[2]   Fania L, Zampetti A, Guerriero G, Feliciani C. Alteration of cholinergic system in keratinocytes cells produces acantholysis: A possible use of cholinergic drugs in pemphigus vulgaris. Antiinflamm Antiallergy Agents Med Chem 2012; 11(3): 238-42.
[http://dx.doi.org/10.2174/1871523011202030238] [PMID: 23140385]

[3]   Namazi MR. Practice pearl: Gargling with cholinergic ophthalmic drops for treating the oral lesions of pemphigus vulgaris. J Drugs Dermatol 2004; 3(5): 484-5.
[PMID: 15552600]

[4]   Gheisari M, Faraji Z, Dadras MS, *et al.* Methylprednisolone pulse therapy plus adjuvant therapy for pemphigus vulgaris: An analysis of 10 years' experience on 312 patients. Dermatol Ther 2019; 32(5):

e13057.
[http://dx.doi.org/10.1111/dth.13057] [PMID: 31400243]

[5]   Jackson S, Gilchrist H, Nesbitt LT Jr. Update on the dermatologic use of systemic glucocorticosteroids. Dermatol Ther 2007; 20(4): 187-205.
[http://dx.doi.org/10.1111/j.1529-8019.2007.00133.x] [PMID: 17970885]

[6]   Chams-Davatchi C, Esmaili N, Daneshpazhooh M, *et al.* Randomized controlled open-label trial of four treatment regimens for pemphigus vulgaris. J Am Acad Dermatol 2007; 57(4): 622-8.
[http://dx.doi.org/10.1016/j.jaad.2007.05.024] [PMID: 17583373]

[7]   Kanwar A, Vinay K. Rituximab in pemphigus. Indian J Dermatol Venereol Leprol 2012; 78(6): 671-6.
[http://dx.doi.org/10.4103/0378-6323.102354] [PMID: 23075635]

CHAPTER 32

Pathergy Testing for Diagnosing Behcet's Disease

Mohammad Reza Namazi[1,*]

[1] *Shiraz University of Medical Sciences and Dr. Namazi Skin and Hair Clinic, Shiraz, Iran*

Behcet's disease (BD) is a type of vasculitis that primarily targets small arteries. According to the International Study Group (ISG) criteria, each major criterion receives two scores: genital aphthous as well as ophthalmic involvements (*i.e.*, retinal vasculitis, anterior uveitis, and posterior uveitis). Each of the minor criterion receives one of the following scores: positive pathergy test, oral aphthous, cutaneous lesions (*e.g.*, pseudofolliculitis, erythema nodosum-like lesions), and vascular lesions (*i.e.*, arterial thrombosis, aneurysm, phlebitis, superficial phlebitis, large vein thrombosis). A total of three or more scores establishes a diagnosis of BD.

The most common manifestation of BD is the presence of recurring, painful mucosal and cutaneous ulcers (> 3 times a year). Many of the manifestations of this syndrome are dermatological, and therefore, dermatologists should know how to perform pathergy tests. A positive pathergy test constitutes one of the diagnostic criteria for BD due to its specificity.

To perform the pathergy test, a thick 20 gauge needle is inserted beveled up into the skin of volar forearm at 45 degrees to a depth of 3-5 mm. The bevel should be concealed under the skin, and some experts suggest the withdrawal of the needle with a rotating movement. Using disinfectants prior to testing is reported to decrease the positivity rate of the test. The site is seen after 48 hours. The presence of an erythematous papule or pustule is considered positive. Erythema without any induration is considered negative. Positive rates can be enhanced by having at least two needle pricks.

Finer needles are unlikely to inflict adequate trauma to reliably induce a pathergy reaction.

Whether the use of corticosteroids interferes in the result of the pathergy test is controversial.

---

[*] **Corresponding author Mohammad Reza Namazi:** Shiraz University of Medical Sciences and Dr. Namazi Skin and Hair Clinic, Shiraz, Iran; E-mail: rezanamazi12@yahoo.com

The papules and pustules resulting from pathergy testing usually become largest in 2 days and vanish within 45 days.

The highest positivity rate for the pathergy test is seen in countries along the Silk Route, *i.e.*, the Middle East, Far East, and Mediterranean Basin.

Pathergy is seen in some other neutrophilic skin diseases, including pyoderma gangrenosum, erythema elevatum diutinum, Sweet syndrome and blind loop syndrome. However, each of these diseases has its specific manifestations and is improbable to be mistaken with BD based on a positive pathergy test [1].

REFERENCE

[1] Rahman S, Daveluy S. Pathergy test. In: StatPearls. Treasure Island: StatPearls Publishing 2022.

CHAPTER 33

Mild-to-Moderate Psoriasis Tips

Alyssa Curcio[1], Christina Kontzias[1] and Steven R. Feldman[1,2,*]

[1] *Center for Dermatology Research, Department of Dermatology, Wake Forest School of Medicine, Winston-Salem, North Carolina, USA*

[2] *Department of Social Sciences & Health Policy, Wake Forest School of Medicine, Winston-Salem, North Carolina, USA*

Psoriasis is a chronic inflammatory condition. Understanding patients' preferences and counseling on lifestyle and skin care practices are essential in achieving positive treatment outcomes. Some clinical pearls for providers on management are included below:

-Primary care physicians can manage mild psoriasis. However, a referral to a dermatologist should be made when there is diagnostic uncertainty, progression to moderate or severe psoriasis, or re-calcitrant disease [1].

-Patients should be made aware that plaque psoriasis is a chronic disease. The goal of the treatment is to achieve disease control rather than cure the disease.

-Topical therapy is the first-line treatment for mild to moderate psoriasis. Adherence to topical therapy is crucial in achieving disease control. Medication adherence can be impacted by numerous factors, including complex treatment plans, dissatisfaction with medication formulation, adverse reactions, forgetfulness, cost, and more [2].

-Patients need to understand how and when to apply topical medication. Patients often misunderstand instructions for use, therefore, providing a handout or other forms of written instructions may be helpful.

-Consider patient preferences for the vehicle and formulation when prescribing topical therapy. For example, patients often favor creams over ointments, as creams have lower adhesiveness, are easily spreadable, and are absorbed quickly [3].

* **Corresponding author Steven R. Feldman:** Department of Social Sciences & Health Policy, Wake Forest School of Medicine, Winston-Salem, North Carolina, USA; E-mail: sfeldman@wakehealth.edu

-If a patient is not using a medication as directed, it is important to address other reasons for poor adherence. (Please see the chapter *"Practical Ways to Improve Patient Adherence"* for more information).

There are several adjuncts to topical and systemic treatment that can be employed in the treatment of psoriasis.

• Providers can counsel patients to avoid smoking and heavy alcohol consumption as both are associated with more severe psoriasis [4].

• Providers may consider recommending weight loss in overweight or obese adults (BMI>25) as weight loss can decrease disease severity and improve quality of life [5 - 8].

• Patients may ask about vitamins or supplements (such as fish oil, selenium, and vitamin D) to improve their psoriasis. Currently, there is not enough evidence to support their use in psoriasis treatment [5, 9].

Providers can counsel patients on daily practices to avoid exacerbating their psoriasis. These include:

• Avoid scratching areas of psoriasis, as this can disrupt the integrity of the skin barrier and increase water loss, thus worsening the symptoms [10].

• Recommend showers over baths. Baths cause increased transepidermal water loss and can lead to increased skin dryness and irritation, further causing bothersome symptoms of itch and flaking [11].

• Limit bathing to one shower or bath daily, which should be less than 5 and 15 minutes, respectively. Ensure patients use cool or warm water (hot water should be avoided). Patients should also avoid using washcloths and loofas as they can irritate skin and worsen psoriasis symptoms. Recommend using unscented bars of soap over liquid soap, as the latter is more drying [12].

• Apply a moisturizer within five minutes of bathing to lock in moisture (creams and ointments work best). All the moisturizers, soaps, and other skincare products should be fragrance-free [12].

-For nail psoriasis, advise patients to keep their nails trimmed, wear gloves when doing wet or manual work, and frequently apply emollient to folds and surfaces of affected nails [13, 14]. Patients should also be counseled to avoid artificial nail use as this can increase the risk of nail separation [14].

-For scalp psoriasis, consider prescribing topical solutions over creams or ointments as a topical solution may appear less greasy in the hair, reducing the need to wash hair frequently. Warn patients that the medication may cause a slight burning or sting, which means the medication is making its way through the hair and onto the scalp (where it is needed to treat their psoriasis). Recommend that patients have assistance while applying the topical solution to their scalp. A partner can divide the hair into sections and apply the medication directly to the scalp. Also, advise against coloring hair, tight hairstyles, or using rollers or curling irons, as these can cause skin irritation and psoriasis flare [15].

-Patients with psoriasis also require screening for comorbid diseases. These include:

• Depression and anxiety: Given the higher rates of depression and anxiety in patients with psoriasis, be mindful of the signs and symptoms and refer to a primary care physician or psychiatrist if necessary [16]. Providers should be aware that the severity of psoriasis does not correlate with the degree of psychosocial impact [17].

• Psoriatic arthritis: It is essential to screen for psoriatic arthritis in psoriasis patients. This can be accomplished by asking about joint pain and stiffness (particularly morning stiffness that lasts >1 hour). Delayed diagnosis of psoriatic arthritis can lead to disease progression and irreversible joint damage [18, 19].

-Psoriasis is often underdiagnosed in Black and Hispanic individuals [20]. Familiarize yourself with the appearance of psoriasis on all Fitzpatrick skin types to properly diagnose psoriasis in more melanated skin.

REFERENCES

[1]   Lebwohl M. Psoriasis. Ann Intern Med 2018; 168(7): 49-64.
       [http://dx.doi.org/10.7326/AITC201804030] [PMID: 29610923]

[2]   Armstrong AW, Aldredge L, Yamauchi PS. Managing patients with psoriasis in the busy clinic. J Cutan Med Surg 2016; 20(3): 196-206.
       [http://dx.doi.org/10.1177/1203475415623508] [PMID: 26712930]

[3]   Stein Gold L, Green L, Dhawan S, Vestbjerg B, Praestegaard M, Selmer J. A phase 3, randomized trial demonstrating the improved efficacy and patient acceptability of fixed dose calcipotriene and betamethasone dipropionate cream. J Drugs Dermatol 2021; 20(4): 420-5.
       [http://dx.doi.org/10.36849/JDD.5653] [PMID: 33852251]

[4]   Griffiths CEM, Armstrong AW, Gudjonsson JE, Barker JNWN. Psoriasis. Lancet 2021; 397(10281): 1301-15.
       [http://dx.doi.org/10.1016/S0140-6736(20)32549-6] [PMID: 33812489]

[5]   Ford AR, Siegel M, Bagel J, *et al.* Dietary recommendations for adults with psoriasis or psoriatic arthritis from the medical board of the national psoriasis foundation: a systematic review. JAMA Dermatol 2018; 154(8): 934-50.
       [http://dx.doi.org/10.1001/jamadermatol.2018.1412] [PMID: 29926091]

[6]   Al-Mutairi N, Nour T. The effect of weight reduction on treatment outcomes in obese patients with psoriasis on biologic therapy: A randomized controlled prospective trial. Expert Opin Biol Ther 2014; 14(6): 749-56.
[http://dx.doi.org/10.1517/14712598.2014.900541] [PMID: 24661040]

[7]   Gisondi P, Del Giglio M, Di Francesco V, Zamboni M, Girolomoni G. Weight loss improves the response of obese patients with moderate-to-severe chronic plaque psoriasis to low-dose cyclosporine therapy: a randomized, controlled, investigator-blinded clinical trial. Am J Clin Nutr 2008; 88(5): 1242-7.
[PMID: 18996858]

[8]   Guida B, Napoleone A, Trio R, *et al.* Energy-restricted, n-3 polyunsaturated fatty acids-rich diet improves the clinical response to immuno-modulating drugs in obese patients with plaque-type psoriasis: A randomized control clinical trial. Clin Nutr 2014; 33(3): 399-405.
[http://dx.doi.org/10.1016/j.clnu.2013.09.010] [PMID: 24120032]

[9]   Pona A, Haidari W, Kolli SS, Feldman SR. Diet and psoriasis. Dermatology Online Journal 2019; 25(2)
[http://dx.doi.org/10.5070/D3252042883]

[10]   Fei C, Xu Y, Cao T, Jiang W, Zou Y, Maibach H. Effect of scratching and friction on human skin in vivo. Skin Res Technol 2021; 27(6): 1049-56.
[http://dx.doi.org/10.1111/srt.13057] [PMID: 33999461]

[11]   Green M, Feschuk AM, Kashetsky N, Maibach HI. "Normal" TEWL-how can it be defined? A systematic review. Exp Dermatol 2022; 31(10): 1618-31.
[http://dx.doi.org/10.1111/exd.14635] [PMID: 35753062]

[12]   8 ways to stop your baths and showers from worsening your psoriasis. American academy of dermatology. Available from: https://www.aad.org/public/diseases/psoriasis/skin-care/baths-showers (Accessed September 1 2022).

[13]   Thomas L, Azad J, Takwale A. Management of nail psoriasis. Clin Exp Dermatol 2021; 46(1): 3-8.
[http://dx.doi.org/10.1111/ced.14314] [PMID: 32741010]

[14]   7 nail-care tips that can reduce nail psoriasis. American academy of dermatology. Available from: https://www.aad.org/public/diseases/psoriasis/skin-care/nail-care (Accessed September 1 2022).

[15]   Hair styling tips that can reduce flares of scalp psoriasis. American acadmy of dermatology. Available from: https://www.aad.org/public/diseases/psoriasis/skin-care/hair-tips (Accessed September 1 2022).

[16]   Kim WB, Jerome D, Yeung J. Diagnosis and management of psoriasis. Can Fam Physician 2017; 63(4): 278-85.
[PMID: 28404701]

[17]   Kimball AB, Jacobson C, Weiss S, Vreeland MG, Wu Y. The psychosocial burden of psoriasis. Am J Clin Dermatol 2005; 6(6): 383-92.
[http://dx.doi.org/10.2165/00128071-200506060-00005] [PMID: 16343026]

[18]   Kavanaugh A, Helliwell P, Ritchlin CT. Psoriatic arthritis and burden of disease: Patient perspectives from the population-based multinational assessment of psoriasis and psoriatic arthritis (MAPP) survey. Rheumatol Ther 2016; 3(1): 91-102.
[http://dx.doi.org/10.1007/s40744-016-0029-z] [PMID: 27747516]

[19]   Haroon M, Gallagher P, FitzGerald O. Diagnostic delay of more than 6 months contributes to poor radiographic and functional outcome in psoriatic arthritis. Ann Rheum Dis 2015; 74(6): 1045-50.
[http://dx.doi.org/10.1136/annrheumdis-2013-204858] [PMID: 24525911]

[20]   Kaufman BP, Alexis AF. Psoriasis in skin of color: Insights into the epidemiology, clinical presentation, genetics, quality-of-life impact, and treatment of psoriasis in non-white racial/ethnic groups. Am J Clin Dermatol 2018; 19(3): 405-23.
[http://dx.doi.org/10.1007/s40257-017-0332-7] [PMID: 29209945]

CHAPTER 34

Severe Psoriasis: Pearls

Mohammad Reza Namazi[1,*]

[1] *Shiraz University of Medical Sciences and Dr. Namazi Skin and Hair Clinic, Shiraz, Iran*

Even with today's potent medications, managing severe psoriasis is not always easy. Some pearls are provided:

-In severe psoriasis, if you choose to prescribe methotrexate, you can start cyclosporine simultaneously, and after 2-3 weeks, cyclosporine can be tapered and discontinued while methotrexate can be continued, as the effect of methotrexate, in contrast to cyclosporine, is not initiated rapidly. Moreover, methotrexate is initiated with a small test dose (less than 10 mg), so you would need to use another fast-acting medication initially to control severe disease.

-If the patient has not responded satisfactorily to the older anti-psoriatic medications and you have tried different TNF-alpha inhibitors, of which, one is better than the others but still not adequately effective, you can add another immunosuppressive, such as cyclosporine or methotrexate, or preferably neotigason, to the TNF-alpha inhibitor to control the disease.

-In the author's experience, in severe patients unresponsive to biologics, a cyclosporine-methotrexate combination can be effective. The side-effect profiles of these agents are different, and therefore, they can be a good combination. This combination has been effective in severe rheumatoid arthritis without a substantial increase in side effects [1].

- Psoriatic plaques have a 4.5-fold higher risk of being colonized by *S. aureus* compared to healthy subjects [2], which can cause septicemia due to the altered skin barrier function in psoriasis.

-When to suspect Staphylococcal septicemia in an erythrodermic psoriasis patient? When the patient becomes tachypneic and looks toxic, consider septicemia seriously. These patients may be afebrile. You see these patients putting a blanket/several blankets on themselves, with their heads under the blanket(s).

* **Corresponding author Mohammad Reza Namazi:** Shiraz University of Medical Sciences and Dr. Namazi Skin and Hair Clinic, Shiraz, Iran; E-mail: rezanamazi12@yahoo.com

Their use of blanket(s) is very noticeable and completely different from other patients. I call this "The Blanket Sign". Take this sign very seriously, though it may be seen as a response to the rapid heat loss through dilated vascular channels in severe erythroderma. This sign is also seen in other serious dermatoses like widespread pemphigus and toxic epidermal necrolysis with impending sepsis.

-Shivering seen in erythrodermic patients is the attempt of the body to combat the loss of heat through the dilated vessels in red skin, and may not be necessarily due to infection.

-Erythrodermic psoriasis patients may be anergic to tuberculin tests. Use QFN-gold (IFN-gamma release assay) if you need to start potent immunosuppressives.

-Try to avoid starting immunosuppressives in patients with erythrodermic psoriatis, as they are prone to sepsis. Start high-dose neotigason (1 mg/kg/d), which rapidly controls the disease. Wet wraps can also be added as a topical therapy.

It should be noted that among immunosuppressives, cyclosporine seems safer in patients at risk of septicemia, as no increase in serious infections has been reported in patients treated with cyclosporine alone [3].

-Cyclosporine inhibits the metabolism of statins, making patients prone to statin-induced rhabdomyolysis. Fluvastatin is very rarely reported to cause rhabdomyolysis and is the best choice in combination with cyclosporine. As cyclosporine increases the serum levels of statin, a trial of decreasing statin dose is suggested. Moreover, checking muscle enzyme levels and asking patients to come if they experience muscular pain is suggested.

-A high sodium diet causes cyclosporine-induced renal dysfunction and hypertension, while high potassium and especially high magnesium diets are protective [4].

-Cyclosporine levels are not routinely checked in dermatological practice, unlike in other specialties. It may be beneficial to check levels in higher doses (> 4mg/kg) or where there has been a poor response [5].

-Skin colonization by *S. aureus* in psoriatic patients, with a consequent alteration of the local microbiota, appears to support the inflammatory pathogenesis of psoriasis by contributing to the alteration in the immune response. As already mentioned, *S. aureus* can also cause septicemia in severe psoriasis. Given the therapeutic effect of bleach bath in atopic dermatitis by decreasing *S. aureus* colonization, with even a greater effect compared to oral antibiotics and mupirocin ointment [6], bleach bath may prove to be of use in psoriasis as well, especially in severe cases at risk of staph septicemia.

REFERENCES

[1]   Tugwell P, Pincus T, Yocum D, *et al.* Combination therapy with cyclosporine and methotrexate in severe rheumatoid arthritis. N Engl J Med 1995; 333(3): 137-42.
      [http://dx.doi.org/10.1056/NEJM199507203330301] [PMID: 7791814]

[2]   Ng CY, Huang YH, Chu CF, Wu TC, Liu SH. Risks for *Staphylococcus aureus* colonization in patients with psoriasis: A systematic review and meta-analysis. Br J Dermatol 2017; 177(4): 967-77.
      [http://dx.doi.org/10.1111/bjd.15366] [PMID: 28160277]

[3]   van de Kerkhof PCM, Nestle FO. Psoriasis. In: Bolognia JL, Schaffer JV, Cerroni L, Eds. Dermatology. 4th ed. China: Elsevier Saunders 2012; p. 154.

[4]   Pere AK, Lindgren L, Tuomainen P, *et al.* Dietary potassium and magnesium supplementation in cyclosporine-induced hypertension and nephrotoxicity. Kidney Int 2000; 58(6): 2462-72.
      [http://dx.doi.org/10.1046/j.1523-1755.2000.00429.x] [PMID: 11115079]

[5]   Jiyad Z, Flohr C. Handbook of Skin Disease Management. 1st ed. India: John Wiley & Sons Ltd. 2023; p. 14.
      [http://dx.doi.org/10.1002/9781119829072.ch7]

[6]   Bath-Hextall FJ, Birnie AJ, Ravenscroft JC, Williams HC. Interventions to reduce Staphylococcus aureus in the management of atopic eczema: An updated Cochrane review. Br J Dermatol 2011; 164(1): 228.
      [http://dx.doi.org/10.1111/j.1365-2133.2010.10078.x] [PMID: 20874857]

Seborrheic Dermatitis Tips

Mohammad Reza Namazi[1,*]

[1] *Shiraz University of Medical Sciences and Dr. Namazi Skin and Hair Clinic, Shiraz, Iran*

Seborrhoeic dermatitis is a common, chronic, or relapsing condition. Dandruff, also called pityriasis capitis, is its uninflamed form . Stress and lack of sleep, immunosuppression, neurological and psychiatric diseases and the use of antipsychotics are the triggering factors [1]. Some interesting tips on seborrheic dermatitis are provided:

- Avoid organic oils, especially olive oil, when treating seborrheic dermatitis or other inflammatory skin diseases triggered by colonizing microflora. Malassezia digests sebum into saturated and unsaturated fatty acids. Saturated fatty acids encourage Malassezia overgrowth, and unsaturated fatty acids induce inflammation and scaling. Organic oils (such as olive oil) contain both saturated and unsaturated lipids and, therefore, may be counterproductive in seborrheic dermatitis. In fact, olive oil is a standard *in vitro* culture medium for Malassezia. As a non-digestible oil, mineral oil may provide a triglyceride-free alternative to organic oils [2].

- Some strains of Malassezia are resistant to azole anti-fungals [1, 3]. Try zinc pyrithione, pyroctone olamine or selenium sulphide instead. Azole anti-fungals contain an azole ring and include clotrimazole, ketoconazole, miconazole, fluconazole, itraconazole, and climbazole. This point should be considered not only in the management of seborrheic dermatitis but also in managing other Malassezia-associated superficial mycoses, such as pityriasis versicolor and Malassezia folliculitis.

* **Corresponding author Mohammad Reza Namazi:** Shiraz University of Medical Sciences and Dr. Namazi Skin and Hair Clinic, Shiraz, Iran; E-mail: rezanamazi12@yahoo.com

REFERENCES

[1]   Dermnet. seborrheic dermatitis. Available from: https://dermnetnz.org/topics/seborrhoeic-dermatitis (Accessed 1/11/2023).

[2]   Siegfried E, Glenn E. Use of olive oil for the treatment of seborrheic dermatitis in children. Arch Pediatr Adolesc Med 2012; 166(10): 967.
[http://dx.doi.org/10.1001/archpediatrics.2012.765] [PMID: 22893193]

[3]   Leong C, Chan JWK, Lee SM, *et al.* Azole resistance mechanisms in pathogenic *M. furfur.* Antimicrob Agents Chemother 2021; 65(5): 01975-20.
[http://dx.doi.org/10.1128/AAC.01975-20] [PMID: 33619053]

CHAPTER 36

Wound Vac and Hyperbaric Oxygen for Wound Healing

Mohammad Reza Namazi[1,*]

[1] *Shiraz University of Medical Sciences and Dr. Namazi Skin and Hair Clinic, Shiraz, Iran*

Negative-pressure wound therapy (NPWT), also known as vacuum-assisted closure (VAC), is a therapeutic technique using a suction pump to remove excess exudate and promote healing in wounds. The therapy involves the controlled application of sub-atmospheric pressure to the wound using a sealed dressing connected to a vacuum pump.

The use of Wound Vac is recommended for the treatment of a range of wounds, including dehisced surgical wounds, pressure ulcers, diabetic foot ulcers, and venous insufficiency ulcers.

NPWT enhances wound healing by removing excess extracellular fluid and decreasing tissue edema, leading to increased blood flow. A decrease in inflammatory mediators, matrix metalloproteinase activity and bacterial burden and an increase in fibroblast proliferation and migration, collagen organization, and expression of vascular endothelial growth factor and fibroblast growth factor-2 are found to occur with this therapy [1].

Oxygen is a crucial component of many biological processes and is necessary for wound healing. Chronic wounds are considered to be hypoxic, with the partial pressure of oxygen in the center of the wound being often below a critical threshold required for the full support of the enzymatic processes necessary for tissue repair [2]. Hyperbaric oxygen therapy consists of using pure oxygen at increased pressure causing enhanced oxygen levels in the blood and tissue. The increased oxygen bioavailability exerts anti-microbial, immunomodulatory and angiogenic properties [3].

In Australia, the author saw an old lady who had a large wound secondary to vasculitis on the back of her right foot, which did not respond to many sessions of

* **Corresponding author Mohammad Reza Namazi:** Shiraz University of Medical Sciences and Dr. Namazi Skin and Hair Clinic, Shiraz, Iran; E-mail: rezanamazi12@yahoo.com

Wound Vac over several months, though vasculitis was well under control. She showed an unbelievably dramatic response to hyperbaric oxygen therapy.

REFERENCES

[1]   Norman G, Shi C, Goh EL, *et al.* Negative pressure wound therapy for surgical wounds healing by primary closure. Cochrane Database Syst Rev 2022; 4(4): CD009261.
[PMID: 35471497]

[2]   Frykberg RG. Topical wound oxygen therapy in the treatment of chronic diabetic foot ulcers. Medicina 2021; 57(9): 917.
[http://dx.doi.org/10.3390/medicina57090917] [PMID: 34577840]

[3]   Sen S, Sen S. Therapeutic effects of hyperbaric oxygen: Integrated review. Med Gas Res 2021; 11(1): 30-3.
[http://dx.doi.org/10.4103/2045-9912.310057] [PMID: 33642335]

CHAPTER 37

Some Tips on Head Lice Management

Mohammad Reza Namazi[1,*]

[1] *Shiraz University of Medical Sciences and Dr. Namazi Skin and Hair Clinic, Shiraz, Iran*

There are several therapeutic options for head lice infestation. A report from India in 1978 demonstrated the efficacy of oral Co-trimoxazole against pediculosis capitis [1]. Some other researchers also claim it to be effective [2]. In contrast to the above reports, a study on 7495 infested Korean children found no benefit in adding co-trimoxazole to lindane shampoo [3]. An Egyptian study in 1996 concluded that a prolonged course of oral co-trimoxazole was needed to free the patients from the adult and nymphal stages but not the eggs (nits) and that until the discovery of a cheap, safe and effective oral drug, topical application of pediculicides was the method of choice [4]. This author's experience does not corroborate the efficacy of co-trimoxacole against pediculosis.

Topical ivermectin lotion has currently been approved by the FDA for the treatment of lice. Oral ivermectin is not FDA-approved. However, in case of patients who are resistant or noncompliant with topical pediculicides, oral ivermectin can be considered. It is highly effective, though resistance is now being reported [5].

The National Health Service (NHS), a publicly funded healthcare system in England, advises that permethrin, electric combs for head lice, and tea tree and plant oils are unlikely to be effective and advises wet combing as the initial management [6]. Details of wet combing can be obtained from the NHS website.

-Advise patients not to use a combination shampoo/conditioner or a conditioner before using lice medicine and not rewash the hair for 1–2 days after the lice medicine is removed [7].

Nits that are attached more than ¼ inch from the base of the hair shaft are almost always hatched (non-viable) [7, 8]. Hatched nits are whitish and collapsed, whereas unhatched nits are dark, round, and translucent, but the best way of differentiation is to examine them for the presence of an operculum, which in-

[*] **Corresponding author Mohammad Reza Namazi:** Shiraz University of Medical Sciences and Dr. Namazi Skin and Hair Clinic, Shiraz, Iran; E-mail: rezanamazi12@yahoo.com

dicates that the nits are unhatched [9]. Importantly, if only hatched nits are seen after treatment, re-treatment is not required [7]. Many flea combs made for cats and dogs are effective for the removal of nits [7].

REFERENCES

[1]   Shashindran CH, Gandhi IS, Krishnasamy S, Ghosh MN. Oral therapy of pediculosis capitis with cotrimoxazole. Br J Dermatol 1978; 98(6): 699-700.
[http://dx.doi.org/10.1111/j.1365-2133.1978.tb03591.x] [PMID: 678457]

[2]   Hipolito RB, Mallorca FG, Zuniga-Macaraig ZO, Apolinario PC, Wheeler-Sherman J. Head lice infestation: Single drug versus combination therapy with one percent permethrin and trimethoprim/sulfamethoxazole. Pediatrics 2001; 107(3): 30.
[http://dx.doi.org/10.1542/peds.107.3.e30] [PMID: 11230611]

[3]   Sim S, Lee IY, Lee KJ, *et al.* A survey on head lice infestation in Korea (2001) and the therapeutic efficacy of oral trimethoprim/sulfamethoxazole adding to lindane shampoo. Korean J Parasitol 2003; 41(1): 57-61.
[http://dx.doi.org/10.3347/kjp.2003.41.1.57] [PMID: 12666731]

[4]   Morsy TA, Ramadan NI, Mahmoud MS, Lashen AH. On the efficacy of Co-trimoxazole as an oral treatment for pediculosis capitis infestation. J Egypt Soc Parasitol 1996; 26(1): 73-7.
[PMID: 8721230]

[5]   Amanzougaghene N, Fenollar F, Raoult D, Mediannikov O. Where are we with human lice? a review of the current state of knowledge. Front Cell Infect Microbiol 2020; 9: 474.
[http://dx.doi.org/10.3389/fcimb.2019.00474] [PMID: 32039050]

[6]   NHS. Head lice and Nits Available from: https://www.nhs.uk/conditions/head-lice-and-nits/ (Accessed /19/2023).

[7]   CDC.Headlice.   2023.   Available   from:
https://www.cdc.gov/parasites/lice/head/diagnosis.html#:~:text=Nits%20that%20are%20attached%20 more,nymph%20inside%20a%20viable%20nit (Accessed /19/2023).

[8]   Namazi MR. Levamisole: A safe and economical weapon against pediculosis. Int J Dermatol 2001; 40(4): 292-4.
[http://dx.doi.org/10.1046/j.1365-4362.2001.01190.x] [PMID: 11454092]

[9]   Namazi MR. Treatment of pediculosis capitis with thiabendazole: A pilot study. Int J Dermatol 2003; 42(12): 973-6.
[http://dx.doi.org/10.1111/j.1365-4632.2003.01996.x] [PMID: 14636196]

CHAPTER 38

Cutaneous Leishmaniasis Pearls

Mohammad Reza Namazi[1,*]

[1] *Shiraz University of Medical Sciences and Dr. Namazi Skin and Hair Clinic, Shiraz, Iran*

Leishmaniasis is seen in approximately 90 countries, however, only scant information on its management is provided in major textbooks.

Cutaneous leishmaniasis (CL) presents as ulcerated/non-ulcerated papules on exposed body parts, which leave unsightly scars. Pentavalent antimony-containing medications, given by intra-muscular injection, are the standard treatments for CL.

Glucantime (made by Sanofi-Aventis, France) comes in 5 cc ampoules having 1500 mg meglumine antimonate equivalent to 405 mg of pentavalent antimony (Sb5+), *i.e.* 81 mg of Sb5+/ ml. It can be injected intra-lesionally in some situations, such as the presence of just a few lesions. The parenteral dose is 20 mg Sb5+/kg/day × 20 days1 [1]. In our experience, the lesions that are partially healed at the end of the treatment continue to be healed for a further 2-3 weeks after discontinuing Glucantime. The approximate volume of Glucantime, which should be injected per day, can be calculated by dividing the patient's weight by 4 (accurately, 4.05), with the maximum volume of injection being 15 cc/d (3 ampoules) [2]. For example, if a patient's weight is 30 kg, 7.5 cc (1.5 ampoules) should be injected per day. Some references recommend using lower doses, *i.e.* 10-20 mg/kg/d [3]. This lower dose may be considered in patients having internal problems, such as cardiac disease.

Glucantime is administered by deep intramuscular injection. If the injection volume is more than 10 ml, it is halved, and each half is injected into each buttock/thigh [4][1].

While the Glucantime brochure states the intramuscular route as the mode of drug administration, some researchers have used the intravenous route, which may be more feasible for some patients [1, 2]. Likewise, the WHO manual mentions both intramuscular and intravenous routes for drug administration. For intravenous ad-

---

[*] **Corresponding author Mohammad Reza Namazi:** Shiraz University of Medical Sciences and Dr. Namazi Skin and Hair Clinic, Shiraz, Iran; E-mail: rezanamazi12@yahoo.com

ministration in adults, Glucantime should be diluted in 50–200 ml of 5% dextrose solution and administered over 0.5-1 hours [4].

According to the WHO manual [4], severe adverse reactions are more likely to be seen in the elderly, while not being absolutely contraindicated. We used Glucantime in patients over 50 years with cardiology consultation prior to the drug administration and twice weekly ECG monitoring without seeing any problem. Also, in the elderly, we used Glucantime in lower doses, even half the usual dose of 20 mg Sb5+/kg/day, and frequently we found it effective.

According to the WHO manual [4], the risk of severe, even lethal, reactions is higher in cases of patients who have heart problems, especially arrhythmia, renal failure or hepatic disorder, serious malnourishment/seriously impaired general condition, advanced HIV, and pregnancy. In these situations, another treatment should be used.

According to the WHO manual [4], patient monitoring is as follows:

• A full blood count is performed prior to and then weekly during the treatment.

• Hepatic function tests are required before and weekly during the treatment. If the level of one of the serum aminotransferases elevates to 3-4 times the upper normal limit, then treatment should be stopped.

• Very rare cases of pancreatitis are reported. However, monitoring of serum amylase and lipase should be done before and weekly during the treatment. If the serum amylase level elevates to more than 4 times the upper normal limit, serum lipase level increases to more than 15 times the upper normal limit, enzyme levels rise rapidly or are accompanied by abdominal pain, nausea and vomiting, the treatment should be temporarily discontinued.

• Very rare cases of acute renal failure are reported. However, renal function tests should be performed before and weekly during the treatment.

• ECG monitoring should be performed twice per week. The most common ECG change is prolonged QT interval, therefore, extreme care should be taken while prescribing Glucantime to patients on drugs that can prolong QT intervals, such as anticholinergics and azithromycin. Other common changes include T inversion, ST depression, and ST elevation. ECG changes are dose-dependent and generally reversible [5].

In the author's experience, topical paramomycin-U is not effective against cutaneous leishmaniasis caused by *L. Tropica* and *L. Major*. While the author was a fellow in the US, Prof. Gil Yosipvitch also pointed out that Israeli researchers have not found it to be effective (G. Yosipovitch, personal communication, May 2008). Clofazimine [6], azithromycin, fluconazole, rifampin, terbinafine, dapsone, hydroxychloroquine, allopurinol, bisphosphonates and proton pump inhibitors, which are claimed to be effective by some researchers, were not found to be very effective in the author's experience, but liposomal amphotericin can be effective on thin lesions.

Interestingly, some clinicians believe that cryotherapy with nitrous oxide is better than that with liquid nitrogen, as the coldness of the former is sufficient to kill the parasite without causing undesirable tissue destruction seen with the latter, with resultant less scar formation[2]. Research on this interesting personal experience is warranted.

Some preventive measures to control leishmaniasis include draining stagnant reservoirs of water, oiling swamps, controlling dogs, destroying the burrows of rodents, plastering houses, cowsheds and latrines using a combination of mud and lime up to a height of 1.22 m, Indoor Residual Spraying (spraying all interior and exterior parts of houses and animal residences with insecticides), planting the noxious plant Bougainvillea glabra, growing attractive plants for sand flies (like Ochradenus baccatus) and using glue traps around them or spraying the sucrose-boric acid mixture on them and spraying the combination of brown sugar, boric acid, and water as an attractive toxic bait on vegetation [7 - 9].

Personal preventive measures for travelers include minimizing the amount of exposed skin by wearing long-sleeved shirts, long pants and socks and tucking the shirts into the pants, applying insect repellent to exposed skin and under the ends of sleeves and pant legs (The most efficacious repellents contain DEET (N,N-diethylmetatoluamide)), spraying living/sleeping places with an insecticide, using a bed net and tucking it under the mattress, considering that sand flies are much tinier than mosquitoes and can pass through smaller holes and using a bed net soaked in/sprayed with a pyrethroid-containing insecticide . The same measures can be employed for screens, curtains, sheets, and clothing (retreating the clothing should be done after 5 washings) [10].

[1] I thank Dr. Maryamsadat Sadati for her helpful comments on Glucantime dosage.

[2] I thank Dr. Masoud Koraee for sharing this pearl.

REFERENCES

[1]   Chrusciak-Talhari A, Dietze R, Talhari S, *et al.* Randomized controlled clinical trial to access efficacy and safety of miltefosine in the treatment of cutaneous leishmaniasis Caused by Leishmania (Viannia) guyanensis in Manaus, Brazil. Am J Trop Med Hyg 2011; 84(2): 255-60.
       [http://dx.doi.org/10.4269/ajtmh.2011.10-0155] [PMID: 21292895]

[2]   Machado PR, Ampuero J, Guimarães LH, *et al.* Miltefosine in the treatment of cutaneous leishmaniasis caused by Leishmania braziliensis in Brazil: A randomized and controlled trial. PLoS Negl Trop Dis 2010; 4(12): 912.
[http://dx.doi.org/10.1371/journal.pntd.0000912] [PMID: 21200420]

[3]   Mohammadzadeh M, Behnaz F, Golshan Z. Efficacy of glucantime for treatment of cutaneous leishmaniasis in Central Iran. J Infect Public Health 2013; 6(2): 120-4.
[http://dx.doi.org/10.1016/j.jiph.2012.11.003] [PMID: 23537825]

[4]   WHO. Draft Manual for case management of cutaneous leishmaniasis in the WHO Eastern Mediterranean Region 2013. http://www.emro.who.int/images/stories/zoonoses/Manual_leishm-aniasis_edited_MB_draft_for_Web_1_5_13.pdf

[5]   Sadeghian G, Ziaei H, Sadeghi M. Electrocardiographic changes in patients with cutaneous leishmaniasis treated with systemic glucantime. Ann Acad Med Singap 2008; 37(11): 916-8.
[http://dx.doi.org/10.47102/annals-acadmedsg.V37N11p916] [PMID: 19082196]

[6]   Namazi MR, Dastgheib L, Mazandarani J, Jowkar F. Clofazimine, an antimycobacterial with potent in vitro and in vivo leishmanicidal activity, is ineffective against cutaneous Leishmania major infection in humans. J Am Acad Dermatol 2010; 62(5): 890-2.
[http://dx.doi.org/10.1016/j.jaad.2009.07.011] [PMID: 20398820]

[7]   Laboudi M, Sahibi H, Elabandouni M, Nhammi H, Ait Hamou S, Sadak A. A review of cutaneous leishmaniasis in Morocco: A vertical analysisto determine appropriate interventions for control and prevention. Acta Trop 2018; 187: 275-83.
[http://dx.doi.org/10.1016/j.actatropica.2018.07.019] [PMID: 30056074]

[8]   Kaldas RM, El Shafey AS, Shehata MG, Samy AM, Villinski JT. Experimental effect of feeding on Ricinus communis and Bougainvillea glabra on the development of the sand fly Phlebotomus papatasi (Diptera: Psychodidae) from Egypt. J Egypt Soc Parasitol 2014; 44(1): 1-12.
[http://dx.doi.org/10.12816/0006441] [PMID: 24961006]

[9]   Coulibaly CA, Traore B, Dicko A, *et al.* Impact of insecticide-treated bednets and indoor residual spraying in controlling populations of Phlebotomus duboscqi, the vector of Leishmania major in Central Mali. Parasit Vectors 2018; 11(1): 345.
[http://dx.doi.org/10.1186/s13071-018-2909-2] [PMID: 29898753]

[10]   Availalble from: https://www.cdc.gov/parasites/leishmaniasis/prevent.html

CHAPTER 39

Alopecia Areata: Some Tips

Mohammad Reza Namazi[1],*

[1] *Shiraz University of Medical Sciences and Dr. Namazi Skin and Hair Clinic, Shiraz, Iran*

Alopecia areata is an autoimmune disease with a strong, complex hereditary component. It is believed that the loss of immune privilege in anagen hair follicles causes the follicle auto-antigens to be presented to auto-reactive CD8+ T cells, with subsequent auto-immune attack of the anagen follicles causing premature transition into telogen phase with ultimate loss of hair [1].

Anthralin is a topical irritant, which is suggested to be effective against alopecia areata, at least partly, through its toxicity to Langerhans cells [2]. Other irritants do not have this effect.

• Patients usually tolerate anthralin better than diphencyprone.

• Topical anthralin is prescribed as: 0.5% anthralin + 2.5% salicylic acid in petrolatum. Salicylic acid prevents the oxidation of anthralin. Petrolatum is the best base for anthralin. The compound is applied on the alopecic patch (or total scalp) as a very thin smear. It should not be massaged on the scalp and should be wiped off once the patient feels burning. The patient should be advised that if the treated area becomes very irritated, he/she can stop applying it for a few days. Loratadine helps with itch. Some experts use a 1% cream applied for 2 hours thrice weekly.

• A disadvantage of anthralin is that it colors the skin, which is not so undesirable for patients and is a sign of adherence to the treatment, which is resolved in a few weeks after its discontinuation. Anthralin can color fabrics as well.

• Anthralin can be used in patients who are unresponsive to intralesional steroids or in children who fear injections. Like other drugs, it may be ineffective in some patients. A randomized controlled study comparing the use of diphencyprone and anthralin in the treatment of extensive chronic alopecia areata showed no statistical difference between the two treatments [3].

---

* **Corresponding author Mohammad Reza Namazi:** Shiraz University of Medical Sciences and Dr. Namazi Skin and Hair Clinic, Shiraz, Iran; E-mail: rezanamazi12@yahoo.com

Interestingly, the author observed some alopecia areata patients disappointed with many treatments who experienced hair re-growth after wearing a wig. Can improvement of the patient's psychological condition and its positive effect on the immune system be responsible?

Some references mention that chronic alopecia areata can end up in scarring alopecia. However, this seems to occur in up to 25% of patients [4], and this author saw an outstanding response to JAK inhibitors in many cases of chronic alopecia areata lasting over 10 years.

The standard dose of tofacitinib is 5 mg BID, but some patients respond to 15 or 20 mg/d. CBC, LFT and Lipids should be checked. CK elevation has no importance. Recurrence on discontinuation is frequent. Baricitinib may have a better safety profile [5].

REFERENCES

[1]   Dermnet. Alopecia areata. Available from: https://dermnetnz.org/topics/alopecia-areata (Accessed 9/26/2022).

[2]   Morhenn VB, Orenberg EK, Kaplan J, Pfendt E, Terrell C, Engleman EG. Inhibition of a Langerhans cell-mediated immune response by treatment modalities useful in psoriasis. J Invest Dermatol 1983; 81(1): 23-7.
       [http://dx.doi.org/10.1111/1523-1747.ep12537586] [PMID: 6863976]

[3]   Rocha VB, Kakizaki P, Donati A, Machado CJ, Pires MC, Contin LA. Randomized controlled study comparing the use of diphencyprone and anthralin in the treatment of extensive chronic alopecia areata. An Bras Dermatol 2021; 96(3): 372-6.
       [http://dx.doi.org/10.1016/j.abd.2020.06.018] [PMID: 33849753]

[4]   Sellheyer K, Bergfeld WF. Histopathologic evaluation of alopecias. Am J Dermatopathol 2006; 28(3): 236-59.
       [http://dx.doi.org/10.1097/00000372-200606000-00051] [PMID: 16778532]

[5]   Vazquez-Herrera NE, Tosti A. Alopecia areata: Clinical treatment. In: Tosti A, Ed. Asz-Sigall D, Pirmes R. Hair and Scalp Treatments. Switzerland: Springer 2020; pp. 109-24.
       [http://dx.doi.org/10.1007/978-3-030-21555-2_9]

CHAPTER 40

The Benefits of Potassium Permanganate

Mohammad Reza Namazi[1,*]

[1] *Shiraz University of Medical Sciences and Dr. Namazi Skin and Hair Clinic, Shiraz, Iran*

Potassium permanganate is a very cheap, oxidizing, astringent, anti-septic, and anti-fungal agent [1] that is beneficial to the infected or weeping wounds and lesions. It helps to resolve the infections and dry the weeping lesions.

-Potassium permanganate does not irritate the wound.

-Patient and clinician education should stress the importance of visual assessment rather than formulaic calculations in the safe preparation of potassium permanganate solution [2]. It is a powder with relatively big grains. The patient should drop a few grains in tap water, preferably boiled, or normal saline and stir the mixture to make a pink or slightly purple solution. Then, he/she should soak a gauze with the solution and apply it to the wound (wet compress). An infected wound on the limb can be directly soaked in potassium permanganate solution made in a big basin as directed above.

-While a pink or slightly purple solution does not color the skin, a dark solution can, which is worrisome to some patients, however, it resolves.

- Adding a small amount of permanganate potassium to a tub of water can be very helpful for the prevention of infection in patients with generalized pemphigus or toxic epidermal necrolysis.

-Topical 5% potassium permanganate solution accelerates healing in chronic diabetic foot ulcers [3].

-*Staphylococcus aureus* skin colonization is correlated with disease severity in atopic dermatitis, suggesting an infection–inflammation cycle. In a Cochrane review of various interventions to reduce *S. aureus* colonization, including oral antibiotics, topical steroids and antibiotic ointments, only bleach bath showed a significant improvement in atopic dermatitis severity [4]. Although bleach bath is

* **Corresponding author Mohammad Reza Namazi:** Shiraz University of Medical Sciences and Dr. Namazi Skin and Hair Clinic, Shiraz, Iran; E-mail: rezanamazi12@yahoo.com

generally well-tolerated, with no existing report on skin irritation, it is usually difficult to ensure patients that a potential irritant is beneficial for sensitive skin, which can significantly undermine their therapeutic adherence despite their apparent acceptance to use it. Potassium permanganate can be an excellent alternative to bleach for this purpose.

REFERENCES

[1]   Burkhart CG, Katz KA. Other topical medications. In: Goldsmith LA, Katz SI, Gilchrest BA, Paller AS, Leffell AJ, Wolf K, Eds. Other topican medications In: Fitzpatrick's Dermatology in General Medicine. 8th ed. USA: McGraw-Hill 2012; pp. 2697-707.

[2]   Chin G, Nicholson H, Demirel S, Affleck A. Topical potassium permanganate solution use in dermatology: Comparison of guidelines and clinical practice. Clin Exp Dermatol 2022; 47(5): 966-7.
[http://dx.doi.org/10.1111/ced.15076] [PMID: 34939207]

[3]   Delgado-Enciso I, Madrigal-Perez VM, Lara-Esqueda A, *et al.* Topical 5% potassium permanganate solution accelerates the healing process in chronic diabetic foot ulcers. Biomed Rep 2018; 8(2): 156-9.
[http://dx.doi.org/10.3892/br.2018.1038] [PMID: 29435274]

[4]   Bath-Hextall FJ, Birnie AJ, Ravenscroft JC, Williams HC. Interventions to reduce Staphylococcus aureus in the management of atopic eczema: An updated Cochrane review. Br J Dermatol 2011; 164(1): 228.
[http://dx.doi.org/10.1111/j.1365-2133.2010.10078.x] [PMID: 20874857]

CHAPTER 41

Strengthening the Immune Response

Mohammad Reza Namazi[1,*]

[1] *Shiraz University of Medical Sciences and Dr. Namazi Skin and Hair Clinic, Shiraz, Iran*

In some skin diseases, like mycosis fungoides, malignant melanoma, genital warts and recurrent herpes, it is beneficial to boost the immune response.

- A paper published in *Nature* reported that Schiff base-forming drugs, including vitamin B6, enhance the CD4 T cell activation by providing a costimulatory signal [1], which has implications in the treatment of the above-mentioned conditions. The no-observed-adverse-effect-level of vitamin B6 is set at 200 mg/d and the safe upper limit at 100 mg/d [2]. Vitamin B6 has the potential to augment the immune response to imiquimod (Please see the chapter "Genital warts: Tips"). Imiquimod enhances Langerhans cell migration from the skin to the draining lymph nodes where Langerhans cells present antigens to the CD4 T cells [3]. By provision of a costimulatory signal, vitamin B6 has the potential to enhance the therapeutic effect of imiquimod.

-Selenium also boosts the immune response [4], and the author had a case of recurrent genital herpes who experienced long-term remission by taking vitamin B6 and selenium.

- Zinc enhances the gene expression of IFN-gamma, supporting the development of cell-mediated immune reactions [5]. Zinc stimulates innate and acquired immunity and its supplementation is shown to reduce COVID-19 in-hospital mortality [6].

- Ganoderma lucidum is a mushroom growing on cut or rotten trees. Ganoderma contains some polysaccharides with an immunostimulative action and some triterpenes having a cytotoxic effect. Ganoderma has antiviral, antibacterial, antioxidant and anticancer effects [7, 8].

-Aloe vera contains some polysaccharide biological response modifiers, which are ligands for pattern recognition receptors and augment the immune response. Bio-

* **Corresponding author Mohammad Reza Namazi:** Shiraz University of Medical Sciences and Dr. Namazi Skin and Hair Clinic, Shiraz, Iran; E-mail: rezanamazi12@yahoo.com

logical response modifiers have been reported to have anti-viral, anti-bacterial, anti-fungal, anti-parasitic, and anti-tumor activities [9, 10].

REFERENCES

[1]   Rhodes J, Chen H, Hall SR, *et al.* Therapeutic potentiation of the immune system by costimulatory Schiff base forming drugs. Nature 1995; 377(6544): 71-5.
[http://dx.doi.org/10.1038/377071a0] [PMID: 7659167]

[2]   Katan MB. Hoeveel vitamine B6 is toxisch? Ned Tijdschr Geneeskd 2005; 149(46): 2545-6.
[PMID: 16320662]

[3]   Carlos ECS, Cristovão GA, Silva AA, Ribeiro BCS, Romana-Souza B. Imiquimod-induced *ex vivo* model of psoriatic human skin *via* interleukin-17A signalling of T cells and Langerhans cells. Exp Dermatol 2022; 31(11): 1791-9.
[http://dx.doi.org/10.1111/exd.14659] [PMID: 36054147]

[4]   Hoffmann PR, Berry MJ. The influence of selenium on immune responses. Mol Nutr Food Res 2008; 52(11): 1273-80.
[http://dx.doi.org/10.1002/mnfr.200700330] [PMID: 18384097]

[5]   Namazi MR. Zinc–levamisole combination: Powerful synergistic immunopotentiation? Med Hypotheses 2006; 66(6): 1253.
[http://dx.doi.org/10.1016/j.mehy.2005.12.009] [PMID: 16434148]

[6]   Olczak-Pruc M, Szarpak L, Navolokina A, *et al.* The effect of zinc supplementation on the course of COVID-19 : A systematic review and meta-analysis. Ann Agric Environ Med 2022; 29(4): 568-74.
[http://dx.doi.org/10.26444/aaem/155846] [PMID: 36583325]

[7]   Kladar NV, Gavarić NS, Božin BN. Ganoderma: Insights into anticancer effects. Eur J Cancer Prev 2016; 25(5): 462-71.
[http://dx.doi.org/10.1097/CEJ.0000000000000204] [PMID: 26317382]

[8]   Cör D, Knez Ž, Knez Hrnčič M. Antitumour, antimicrobial, antioxidant and antiacetylcholinesterase effect of ganoderma lucidum terpenoids and polysaccharides: A review. Molecules 2018; 23(3): 649.
[http://dx.doi.org/10.3390/molecules23030649] [PMID: 29534044]

[9]   Leung MYK, Liu C, Koon JCM, Fung KP. Polysaccharide biological response modifiers. Immunol Lett 2006; 105(2): 101-14.
[http://dx.doi.org/10.1016/j.imlet.2006.01.009] [PMID: 16554097]

[10]   Feily A, Namazi MR. Aloe vera in dermatology: A brief review. G Ital Dermatol Venereol 2009; 144(1): 85-91.
[PMID: 19218914]

CHAPTER 42

Macular Amyloidosis Pearls

Mohammad Reza Namazi[1,*]

[1] Shiraz University of Medical Sciences and Dr. Namazi Skin and Hair Clinic, Shiraz, Iran

Macular amyloidosis (MA) is a primary localised cutaneous amyloidosis, where the deposition of amyloid, a proteinaceous material, causes hyperpigmented patches in the skin. There is no standard, very effective treatment for MA [1].

Advise the patients not to massage the area, not to use an exfoliating washcloth, and to avoid tight clothes.

Interestingly, the itch due to MA usually responds to cetirizine.

The following compound gives some beneficial lightening effects in MA:

20% Adapalene (or Tretinoin) cream in Mometasone cream; Qhs application (not massaged on the skin).

As curcumin can both inhibit the formation and promote the disaggregation of amyloid-β plaques in Alzheimer's disease [2], it may also be effective in MA, though the depositions are not exactly the same. My experience with a few cases supports this notion, though meticulous studies should be performed on this subject. It is generally a safe treatment.

REFERENCES

[1]   Maddison B, Namazi MR, Samuel LS, *et al.* Unexpected diminished innervation of epidermis and dermoepidermal junction in lichen amyloidosus. Br J Dermatol 2008; 159(2): 403-6.
[http://dx.doi.org/10.1111/j.1365-2133.2008.08685.x] [PMID: 18547301]

[2]   Tang M, Taghibiglou C. The mechanisms of action of curcumin in Alzheimer's disease. J Alzheimers Dis 2017; 58(4): 1003-16.
[http://dx.doi.org/10.3233/JAD-170188] [PMID: 28527218]

* **Corresponding author Mohammad Reza Namazi:** Shiraz University of Medical Sciences and Dr. Namazi Skin and Hair Clinic, Shiraz, Iran; E-mail: rezanamazi12@yahoo.com

CHAPTER 43

Mycosis Fungoides Pearls

Mohammad Reza Namazi[1,*]

[1] *Shiraz University of Medical Sciences and Dr. Namazi Skin and Hair Clinic, Shiraz, Iran*

Mycosis fungoides (MF), the most common type of primary cutaneous T-cell lymphoma, is characterised by progression from patches to plaques to tumours. While the retinoid-X-receptor-selective bexarotene is the only topical retinoid approved for MF, other retinoids, such as tretinoin, have also been used [1].

-The following compound formulation can be used for MF, especially in resource-limited areas:

20-30% adapalen cream (or tretinoin cream) in mometasone cream.

In this formulation, retinoid increases the penetration of the steroid. Steroid-associated skin atrophy and retinoid-associated irritation can be mitigated by other agents. Moreover, the use of topical steroids can provide additive benefits in conjunction with retinoids for the treatment of MF.

-A good but frequently underutilized option for treating MF is methotrexate [2].

-Importantly, even if the cutaneous lesions are under control, MF patients need lymph node examination in each follow-up. The author has seen controlled MF patients complicated by lymphoma, and Huang *et al.*'s paper [3] also supports this experience.

* **Corresponding author Mohammad Reza Namazi:** Shiraz University of Medical Sciences and Dr. Namazi Skin and Hair Clinic, Shiraz, Iran; E-mail: rezanamazi12@yahoo.com

REFERENCES

[1]   Aires D, Shaath T, Fraga G, Rajpara A, Fischer R, Liu D. Safe and efficacious use of a topical retinoid under occlusion for the treatment of mycosis fungoides. J Drugs Dermatol 2014; 13(12): 1479-80.
[PMID: 25607792]

[2]   Alenezi F, Girard C, Bessis D, Guillot B, Du-Thanh A, Dereure O. Benefit/risk ratio of low-dose methotrexate in cutaneous lesions of mycosis fungoides and Sézary syndrome. Acta Derm Venereol 2021; 101(2): adv00384.
[http://dx.doi.org/10.2340/00015555-3719] [PMID: 33313939]

[3]   Huang KP, Weinstock MA, Clarke CA, McMillan A, Hoppe RT, Kim YH. Second lymphomas and other malignant neoplasms in patients with mycosis fungoides and Sezary syndrome: evidence from population-based and clinical cohorts. Arch Dermatol 2007; 143(1): 45-50.
[http://dx.doi.org/10.1001/archderm.143.1.45] [PMID: 17224541]

CHAPTER 44

The Pro-oxidant Activity of Anti-oxidants and its Practical Implications

Mohammad Reza Namazi[1,*]

[1] *Shiraz University of Medical Sciences and Dr. Namazi Skin and Hair Clinic, Shiraz, Iran*

Anti-oxidants, either topical or ingestible, are one of the most commonly used agents.

Surprisingly, some popular anti-oxidants have been reported to have pro-oxidant behavior. The presence of metal ions, the concentration of the anti-oxidant and its redox potential can affect the pro-oxidant function of the anti-oxidants [1].

-In a paper published in Nature, researchers discovered that while some markers for DNA damage mediated by oxygen radicals decreased, some markers, which were mutagenic, increased in the peripheral blood lymphocytes of volunteers who took a 500 mg/d vitamin C supplement, refuting the notion that vitamin C functions only as an anti-oxidant. However, the authors concluded that at doses less than 500 mg per day, the anti-oxidant effect of vitamin C may predominate [2].

-Vitamin E is also known as a potent anti-oxidant and harmful pro-oxidant at high concentrations. When reacting with reactive oxygen species, it becomes a free radical itself, and if there is not enough vitamin C for its regeneration, it remains in the reactive state [1].

-In conclusion, it is false to consider that the popular anti-oxidants exert just antioxidant activity. Based on their dose and other factors mentioned above, systemically administered anti-oxidants can also demonstrate pro-oxidant effects. This can be true for their topical preparations as well, debunking the claims of some companies about the beneficial effects of their topical vitamin C or vitamin E preparations on the skin without conducting experimental studies.

---

[*] **Corresponding author Mohammad Reza Namazi:** Shiraz University of Medical Sciences and Dr. Namazi Skin and Hair Clinic, Shiraz, Iran; E-mail: rezanamazi12@yahoo.com

REFERENCES

[1]   Sotler R, Poljšak B, Dahmane R. Prooxidant activities of antioxidants and their impact on health. Acta Clin Croat 2019; 58(4): 726-36.
[http://dx.doi.org/10.20471/acc.2019.58.04.20] [PMID: 32595258]

[2]   Podmore ID, Griffiths HR, Herbert KE, Mistry N, Mistry P, Lunec J. Vitamin C exhibits pro-oxidant properties. Nature 1998; 392(6676): 559.
[http://dx.doi.org/10.1038/33308] [PMID: 9560150]

CHAPTER 45

How to Prevent the Growth of Neurofibromas?

Mohammad Reza Namazi[1,*]

¹ Shiraz University of Medical Sciences and Dr. Namazi Skin and Hair Clinic, Shiraz, Iran

Neurofibromas are nerve-sheath tumors composed of Schwann cells, fibroblasts, mast cells, and vascular components. Neurofibromas gradually enlarge, causing cosmetic and functional problems.

-Histamine stimulates fibroblasts to produce more collagen [1]. Many neurofibromatosis patients experience pruritus, which precedes the enlargement of the lesions. Ketotifen, an anti-histamine and mast-cell stabilizer, can be used to prevent the growth of neurofibromas.

-A recent *in vitro* study has shown that hydroxychloroquine can hamper the growth of neurofibromas by enhancing the expression of matrix metalloproteinase 1 [2]. This study awaits clinical trials.

REFERENCES

[1]   Murota H, Bae S, Hamasaki Y, Maruyama R, Katayama I. Emedastine difumarate inhibits histamine-induced collagen synthesis in dermal fibroblasts. J Investig Allergol Clin Immunol 2008; 18(4): 245-52.
        [PMID: 18714531]

[2]   Yumine A, Tsuji G. Hydroxychloroquine induces matrix metalloproteinase 1 expression and apoptosis in neurofibromatosis type 1 Schwann cells. J Dermatol Sci 2021; 104(2): 142-5.
        [http://dx.doi.org/10.1016/j.jdermsci.2021.09.009] [PMID: 34763989]

* **Corresponding author Mohammad Reza Namazi:** Shiraz University of Medical Sciences and Dr. Namazi Skin and Hair Clinic, Shiraz, Iran; E-mail: rezanamazi12@yahoo.com

CHAPTER 46

How to Expedite Depigmentation Therapy in Vitiligo?

Mohammad Reza Namazi[1,*]

[1] *Shiraz University of Medical Sciences and Dr. Namazi Skin and Hair Clinic, Shiraz, Iran*

De-pigmentation therapy is considered for patients with widespread but incomplete vitiligo to improve their appearance. The most commonly used depigmenting agent is monobenzyl ether of hydroquinone (MBEH). De-pigmentation therapy may take several months to produce acceptable results.

The increased activity of inducible nitric oxide synthase (iNOS) has been suggested to be potentially linked to the increased levels of nitric oxide (NO) in vitiligo, leading to the death of melanocytes. Animal studies have shown that L-arginine, the precursor of NO, plays a key role in promoting the effect of MBEH [1]. Therefore, prescribing L-arginine tablets can expedite the depigmentation treatment.

Some studies have shown that proton pump inhibitors can exacerbate vitiligo [2] by rendering melanocytes prone to apoptosis [3]. Therefore, another option could be adding these agents, like lansoprazole, to MBEH therapy. The corollary of this point is that proton pump inhibitors should be avoided in vitiligo patients who are being treated for re-pigmentation.

REFERENCES

[1]   Mansourpour H, Ziari K, Kalantar Motamedi S, Hassan Poor A. Therapeutic effects of iNOS inhibition against vitiligo in an animal model. Eur J Transl Myol 2019; 29(3): 8383.
[http://dx.doi.org/10.4081/ejtm.2019.8383] [PMID: 31579486]

[2]   Holla A, Kumar R, Parsad D, Kanwar AJ. Proton pump inhibitor induced depigmentation in vitiligo. J Cutan Aesthet Surg 2011; 4(1): 46-7.
[http://dx.doi.org/10.4103/0974-2077.79193] [PMID: 21572683]

[3]   Namazi MR. Proton pump inhibitors may trigger vitiligo by rendering melanocytes prone to apoptosis. Br J Dermatol 2008; 158(4): 844-5.
[http://dx.doi.org/10.1111/j.1365-2133.2007.08406.x] [PMID: 18205862]

* **Corresponding author Mohammad Reza Namazi:** Shiraz University of Medical Sciences and Dr. Namazi Skin and Hair Clinic, Shiraz, Iran; E-mail: rezanamazi12@yahoo.com

The Problem in Diagnosing Early Vitiligo

Mohammad Reza Namazi[1,*]

[1] *Shiraz University of Medical Sciences and Dr. Namazi Skin and Hair Clinic, Shiraz, Iran*

While it is mentioned in textbooks that vitiligo demonstrates chalky-white accentuation under Wood's light, early-onset vitiligo shows an off-white accentuation. This causes difficulty in distinguishing vitiligo, especially the segmental type which is more stable than common vitiligo, from nevus depigmentosus.

Nevus depigmentosus (ND), which should correctly be named as nevus hypopigmentosus as it is not depigmented, may not be congenital and can occur after birth, hence presenting as a differential diagnosis for early-onset vitiligo.

Biopsy is not always helpful in confirming vitiligo, as a vitiligo patch is not always devoid of melanocytes, and also the melanin pigmentation may remain for a period of time after the development of vitiligo.

ND has a serrated, irregular margin and has inner pigmentation. It rarely has poliosis. In contrast, vitiligo has a straight border and the inner pigmentation is follicular. ND tends to have a greater vertical width (involving more dermatomes) than vitiligo [1].

REFERENCES

[1]   Roh D, Shin K, Kim WI, *et al.* Clinical differences between segmental nevus depigmentosus and segmental vitiligo. J Dermatol 2019; 46(9): 777-81.
        [http://dx.doi.org/10.1111/1346-8138.15015] [PMID: 31342527]

* **Corresponding author Mohammad Reza Namazi:** Shiraz University of Medical Sciences and Dr. Namazi Skin and Hair Clinic, Shiraz, Iran; E-mail: rezanamazi12@yahoo.com

CHAPTER 48

Vitiligo Pearls

Mohammad Reza Namazi[1,*]

[1] *Shiraz University of Medical Sciences and Dr. Namazi Skin and Hair Clinic, Shiraz, Iran*

Hafez Shirazi, a great Persian poet, said:

"Who is in me, heart-weary, now I know not

While I am mute, a sound within me roars…"

This poem elegantly describes the condition of people suffering from autoimmune diseases. Vitiligo is an autoimmune disorder affecting 1% of the world population [1]. Treatment of this condition is challenging.

Psoralen UVA (PUVA) can be given as PUVAsol (solar irradiation as the source of UVA) [2]:

PUVA-sol is especially useful for patients who cannot visit the hospital frequently and those with economic problems.

For using PUVA-Sol, the author recommends either the compound 20% methoxsalene solution 5% in clobetasol cream or the compound 20% methoxsalene solution 5% + 20% propylene glycol in Alcohol 70° (the compounds have 1% methoxsalen). The topical is applied to the area every other day, and after 0.5-1 hr, the area is exposed to the light passing through a window (UVA) for 20 seconds. The area is then washed, sunscreen is applied and further sun exposure is limited. The exposure time is increased by 10 seconds in each session until a mild erythema is developed. Then, the time is kept constant until an increase is required to maintain the erythema. The best time of exposure is between 11 am to 2 pm. The patient is advised to follow the instructions carefully as this treatment may cause burns. No response after 6 months is considered as failure.

Intralesional tetracosactide, believed to exert MSH-like activity, is not effective against vitiligo in this author's experience.

[*] **Corresponding author Mohammad Reza Namazi:** Shiraz University of Medical Sciences and Dr. Namazi Skin and Hair Clinic, Shiraz, Iran; E-mail: rezanamazi12@yahoo.com

Exposure to the sun is beneficial for vitiligo, but sunburn should be avoided as it can cause the Koebner phenomenon.

Some clinicians prescribe selenium supplements for vitiligo patients, as selenium is an anti-oxidant. However, a meta-analysis showed no significant difference in serum selenium levels between vitiligo patients and healthy controls [3]. Another meta-analysis showed that higher serum selenium and lower zinc levels can increase the risk of vitiligo [4].

Copper levels are significantly higher in vitiligo patients compared to controls [4]. Therefore, though copper induces melanogenesis, its use is not recommended.

Though many believe that hydrogen peroxide is crucially involved in the pathogenesis of vitiligo, de-pigmentation is not reported as a feature of acatalasemia, a condition characterized by high hydrogen peroxide levels due to very low levels of catalase. Interestingly, many people with acatalasemia never experience any health problems [5].

In this author's experience, Vitix gel, claimed by the manufacturer to contain the anti-oxidant enzymes superoxide dismutase and catalase, is not effective against vitiligo. Other researchers have also reached this conclusion [6].

Omega-3 fatty acids inhibit pro-inflammatory cytokines and increase the activity of glutathione peroxidase, an anti-oxidant enzyme that is decreased in vitiligo [7]. Omega-3 fatty acids can help against vitiligo. Clinical trials on this subject are warranted.

Vitiligo patients should be advised to avoid massage and the use of an exfoliating washcloth (to prevent the Koebner phenomenon).

Interestingly, vitiligo may be associated with pruritus in around 20% of cases [8], and scratching the skin can trigger vitiligo (Koebner phenomenon). Therefore, vitiligo patients should be enquired about itch and receive treatment if needed.

Both 5-FU and microneedling are found to accelerate melanocyte migration in vitiligo. They can be combined to produce a stronger effect [9]. 5-FU may also be compounded with topical steroids, *e.g.* , 2% salicylic acid + 2% lactic acid + 40% Efudix cream 5% + mometasone cream qs $\neq$ 60 gr (salicylic acid and lactic acid increase the penetration of other agents by dissolving the horny layer. qs means 'add as much of this ingredient as is needed'; in this formula, 46% of the compound consists of mometasone cream. This topical can be applied BD to compensate for the decreased concentrations of the active ingredients).

Excimer laser is equally efficacious to NBUVB [10].

Tofacitinib 5 mg/d is reported to be effective. Results are enhanced with concurrent NBUVB [10]. The author has seen dramatic results with baricitinib.

- Some expert clinicians use the compound 50% mometasone in isopropyl alcohol for vitiligo, as isopropyl alcohol dramatically increases the penetration of mometasone. Also, the penetration of tarolimus can dramatically be enhanced by propylene glycol, *e.g.* , in the following compound: 10% propylene glycol in tacrolimus cream $\neq$ 60 gr.

REFERENCES

[1]   Namazi MR. What is the important practical implication of detecting decreased G6PD levels in vitiligo? Adv Biomed Res 2015; 4(1): 89.
[http://dx.doi.org/10.4103/2277-9175.156653] [PMID: 26015915]

[2]   Kc S, Karn D. Practical aspects in topical puvasol in dermatology: An experience in a teaching hospital. Kathmandu Univ Med J 2014; 12(48): 306-7.
[PMID: 26333590]

[3]   Dai T, Xiaoying S, Li X, Hongjin L, Yaqiong Z, Bo L. Selenium level in patients with vitiligo: A meta-analysis. BioMed Res Int 2020; 2020: 1-7.
[http://dx.doi.org/10.1155/2020/7580939] [PMID: 32626761]

[4]   Huo J, Liu T, Huan Y, Li F, Wang R. Serum level of antioxidant vitamins and minerals in patients with vitiligo, a systematic review and meta-analysis. J Trace Elem Med Biol 2020; 62: 126570.
[http://dx.doi.org/10.1016/j.jtemb.2020.126570] [PMID: 32593085]

[5]   Available from: https://medlineplus.gov/genetics/condition/acatalasemia/

[6]   Yuksel EP, Aydin F, Senturk N, Canturk T, Turanli AY. Comparison of the efficacy of narrow band ultraviolet B and narrow band ultraviolet B plus topical catalase-superoxide dismutase treatment in vitiligo patients. Eur J Dermatol 2009; 19(4): 341-4.
[http://dx.doi.org/10.1684/ejd.2009.0699] [PMID: 19467974]

[7]   Namazi MR, Chee Leok GOH. Vitiligo and diet: A theoretical molecular approach with practical implications. Indian J Dermatol Venereol Leprol 2009; 75(2): 116-8.
[http://dx.doi.org/10.4103/0378-6323.48654] [PMID: 19293496]

[8]   Vachiramon V, Onprasert W, Harnchoowong S, Chanprapaph K. Prevalence and clinical characteristics of itch in vitiligo and its clinical significance. BioMed Res Int 2017; 2017: 1-8.
[http://dx.doi.org/10.1155/2017/5617838] [PMID: 28828385]

[9]   Albalat W, Elsayed M, Salem A, Ehab R, Fawzy M. Microneedling and 5-flurouracil can enhance the efficacy of non-cultured epidermal cell suspension transplantation for resistant acral vitiligo. Dermatol Ther 2022; 35(10): 15768.
[http://dx.doi.org/10.1111/dth.15768] [PMID: 36190004]

[10]   Jiyad Z, Flohr C. Handbook of Skin Disease Management. 1st ed. India: John Wiley & Sons Ltd. 2023; p. 174.
[http://dx.doi.org/10.1002/9781119829072]

CHAPTER 49

Tips to Prevent Hair Damage

Mohammad Reza Namazi[1,*]

[1] *Shiraz University of Medical Sciences and Dr. Namazi Skin and Hair Clinic, Shiraz, Iran*

Thermal, chemical and mechanical stress can cause trichoptilosis (hair split ends). Examples include the excessive use of hair dryers and curling irons, hair coloring, hair straightening (relaxing), repeated combing and pulling a comb forcefully through the tangled hair. Bleaching is especially very damaging to hair.

Plastic combs, in contrast to wooden combs, produce static electricity, which is harmful to hair.

For the prevention of hair damage, the following points should be recommended to patients [1]:

• Do not relax bleached hair, as it may break.

• Be sure that only the hair root is re-treated if the hair is already relaxed or permanently waved (Hair straightening is repeated every 3-6 months).

• Do not shampoo for at least 3 days after permanent relaxing or waving.

•Always undergo permanent waving or relaxing first and wait for at least 2 weeks before dying the hair.

• Dye hair within its natural color or darker.

Conditioners affect hair shafts by increasing shine, decreasing electricity, improving hair strength, and protecting against UV radiation [1].

Cinere Intense Hair Repair is a leave-on product made by the Iranian company Cinere, containing cationic polymers that provide protection and gloss to the hair by covering the hair and neutralizing the negative electricity charges on it. Its silicone ingredient also provides protection, gloss and softness to the hair and eases combing.

* **Corresponding author Mohammad Reza Namazi:** Shiraz University of Medical Sciences and Dr. Namazi Skin and Hair Clinic, Shiraz, Iran; E-mail: rezanamazi12@yahoo.com

Coconut oil has a high affinity for hair proteins, and due to its low molecular weight and straight linear chain, it is able to penetrate inside the hair shaft, reducing protein loss and preventing hair damage [2].

20 Amp. Vit E in coconut oil # 200 gr, applied after showering on hair ends, miraculously improves damaged hair[1]. The hair should not be massaged with it as massage is traumatic to hair.

[1] I learnt this formula from Dr. Monouchehr Sodaifi, Founding Chair of Dermatology Department of Shiraz University of Medical Sciences, Shiraz, Iran.

REFERENCES

[1]   Gavazzoni Dias MFR. How to Select a Good Shampoo and Conditioner. In: Tosti A, Asz-Sigall D, Pirmez R. Hair and Scalp Treatments, A Practical Guide. Switzerland: Springer; 2020: p. 253-264.

[2]   Rele AS, Mohile RB. Effect of mineral oil, sunflower oil, and coconut oil on prevention of hair damage. J Cosmet Sci 2003; 54(2): 175-92.
[PMID: 12715094]

CHAPTER 50

Androgenetic Hair Loss: Some Important Management Tips

Mohammad Reza Namazi[1,*]

[1] *Shiraz University of Medical Sciences and Dr. Namazi Skin and Hair Clinic, Shiraz, Iran*

Hair loss can inflict significant psychological trauma on patients and is one of the commonest complaints encountered by dermatologists.

Commercial products containing both minoxidil and 5-alpha-reductase inhibitors are not available everywhere, and therefore, should be made by local pharmacists for cases of severe hair loss. The formulations of two topical anti-hair loss compounds are provided:

• 2-5% minoxidil (powder) + 0.0.5%-5% estradiol valerate (powder) + 0.02-0.1% betamethasone (powder) + 5% propylene glycol in Alcohol 70°.

• 2-5% minoxidil (powder) + 5-10% azelaic acid (powder) + 0.02-0.1% betamethasone (powder) + 5% propylen glycol in Alcohol 70°.

Propylene glycol increases the penetration of other agents. Azelaic acid has an anti-androgenic effect. Minoxidil is used in some commercial products like Xandrox in 12.5% concentration, so you can increase its concentration in your formulation if your pharmacist has enough expertise to make the compound. Betamethasone prevents the possible irritation of propylene glycol.

The above formulation, without estradiol/azelaic acid, can be used for telogen effluvium.

Patients may have better compliance with high-concentration topicals once daily than with low-concentration topicals twice daily, perhaps with the same therapeutic effect. A study has shown 5% minoxidil foam once daily to have an efficacy similar to 2% minoxidil solution twice daily [1].

* **Corresponding author Mohammad Reza Namazi:** Shiraz University of Medical Sciences and Dr. Namazi Skin and Hair Clinic, Shiraz, Iran; E-mail: rezanamazi12@yahoo.com

Importantly, in contrast to what the minoxidil brochure states, anti-hair loss solutions should not be massaged on the scalp, as massage can induce telogen effluvium.

Though the anti-androgens, cyproterone acetate, spironolactone, and finasteride, are commonly used in the treatment of hyperandrogenism, flutamide, due to its high potency in blocking testosterone and dihydrotestosterone receptors, is a key drug for this condition. Flutamide comes in 250 mg tablets. An ultra-low dose of 62.5 mg/d was found to be enough to provide anti-androgenic benefits more than the effects jointly conferred by metformin, pioglitazone, and/or estroprogestagens. These benefits included normalizing lipid profiles, circulating androgens, adiponectin, and total body, abdominal, and visceral adiposities [2]. Hepatotoxicity is a rare but potentially fatal side effect of flutamide. Most cases of severe hepatotoxicity were observed when flutamide was given in high doses of 750-1500 mg/d for the management of prostate cancer [2, 3]. Several studies have shown no increase in transaminase levels with low- and ultra-low doses of flutamide, *i.e.*, 125 mg/d and 62.5 mg/d, respectively. However, genetic and ethnic factors seem to play a role in affecting metabolizing enzymes. An Italian study showed mild hypertransaminasemia and rare hepatotoxicity associated with both low- and ultra-low doses of flutamide, with no relationship to the low or ultra-low dose regimens and co-administration of oral contraceptives. Hypertransaminasemia occurred early, with a median time of 12 weeks (range: 2–48). A significant correlation was observed between hepatotoxicity and pretreatment BMI and basal ALT and AST levels. All the patients revealed normalization of AST/ALT levels 4 weeks after the discontinuation of therapy [3, 4]. Therefore, low and ultra-low doses of flutamide can be considered for severe androgenic hair loss, resistant hirsutism, resistant acne, and hidradenitis suppurativa in women. Surveillance of patients, especially at the beginning of the treatment is advisable. Serum transaminase levels should be measured prior to starting the treatment and then measured monthly for the first 4 months of therapy and periodically thereafter. Liver function tests should also be performed at the first signs and symptoms suggestive of liver dysfunction [5] Bicalutamide appears to have lower risks of hepatotoxicity compared to flutamide.

Finasteride Tips:

• There are no data demonstrating the efficacy or safety of finasteride in children under the age of 18 [6].

• Patients on finasteride should not donate blood in order to prevent pregnant women from receiving it with blood transfusion [7].

• Evidence for post-finasteride syndrome (persistent sexual and neurologic side effects) is limited, but this should be explained to patients, otherwise, they may become aware of it by searching the internet and will avoid treatment. Some experts do not prescribe finasteride for patients having a history of depression [6], while some monitor the patients for psychiatric symptoms.

• Gynecomastia is rare but may persist for a long time after drug interruption [7].

• Finasteride does not affect the fertility of young healthy men but should not be given to those with fertility or semen analysis problems [7].

• Prostate-specific antigen levels (PSA) are approximately halved with finasteride 1 mg/d, which can mask the detection of prostate cancer. Therefore, in men over 50 years, checking PSA levels before treatment is suggested [7].

• The efficacy of finasteride in women is not well established, but some studies have shown its efficacy at 2.5-5 mg/d in both pre- and post-menopausal women [7]. 1 mg/d dosage is found to be ineffective against hair loss in postmenopausal women [8].

• Though there is a lack of data showing the link between finasteride and breast cancer, some experts avoid prescribing it for women with personal or family history of breast cancer [7].

Spironolactone (100-200 mg/d) can be used for female pattern hair loss. Starting at 50 mg/d and gradually increasing the dose is recommended. In doses over 100 mg/d, avoidance of potassium intake and monitoring potassium levels are suggested. In sexually active women, it should be prescribed with an OCP, which can preferably contain anti-androgenic agents cyproterone acetate, drospirenone, or dienogest [7]. Spironolactone was not associated with any increased cancer risk in a meta-analysis of over 4.5 million consumers [9].

As flutamide, finasteride, and spironolactone act at different pathophysiologic points of androgenic alopecia, their combinations in resistant or very severe cases deserve consideration.

For managing androgenetic alopecia, PRP+microneedling is suggested to be done for 3 sessions at 1.5- to 2-month intervals. Dutasteride mesotherapy is done every 3 months [10].

Topical minoxidil is compatible with breastfeeding [10].

Low-dose oral minoxidil, *i.e.*, 0.25 mg/d, is found to be effective and well tolerated [10].

Dutasteride (0.5 mg/d) is approved for androgenetic alopecia in some countries. It is more effective than finasteride, with probably similar side effects. A case series has shown it to be effective in cases unresponsive to finasteride [11]. A randomized study on 12 male volunteers showed that dutasteride, but not finasteride, is associated with increased intrahepatic lipid accumulation [12]. A more recent publication has raised the concern that both finasteride and dutasteride may result in non-alcoholic fatty liver disease, insulin resistance and dry eye disease [13]. This issue needs further investigation.

REFERENCES

[1] Blume-Peytavi U, Hillmann K, Dietz E, Canfield D, Garcia Bartels N. A randomized, single-blind trial of 5% minoxidil foam once daily versus 2% minoxidil solution twice daily in the treatment of androgenetic alopecia in women. J Am Acad Dermatol 2011; 65(6): 1126-34.
[http://dx.doi.org/10.1016/j.jaad.2010.09.724] [PMID: 21700360]

[2] de Zegher F, Ibáñez L. Flutamide for androgen excess: Low dose is best. J Pediatr Adolesc Gynecol 2011; 24(2): 43-4.
[http://dx.doi.org/10.1016/j.jpag.2010.02.005] [PMID: 21376280]

[3] Bruni V, Peruzzi E, Dei M, *et al.* Hepatotoxicity with low- and ultralow-dose flutamide: A surveillance study on 203 hyperandrogenic young females. Fertil Steril 2012; 98(4): 1047-52.
[http://dx.doi.org/10.1016/j.fertnstert.2012.06.018] [PMID: 22795685]

[4] Karaahmet F, Kurt K. Hepatotoxicity with flutamide. Fertil Steril 2012; 98(5): 27.
[http://dx.doi.org/10.1016/j.fertnstert.2012.08.045] [PMID: 22985946]

[5] Product Monograph. 2019. Available from: https://www.aapharma.ca/downloads/en/PIL/2019/Flutamide-Pr_Mono_ENG-Mar_7_2019.pdf

[6] Available from: https://www.medicines.org.uk/emc/product/7068/smpc#gref

[7] Kelly Y, Tosti A. Androgenetic Alopecia: Clinical Treatment.Asz-Sigall D, Pirmez R Hair and Scalp Treatments, A practical Guide. Switzerland: Springer 2020; pp. 91-108.
[http://dx.doi.org/10.1007/978-3-030-21555-2_8]

[8] Mysore V, Shashikumar BM. Guidelines on the use of finasteride in androgenetic alopecia. Indian J Dermatol Venereol Leprol 2016; 82(2): 128-34.
[http://dx.doi.org/10.4103/0378-6323.177432] [PMID: 26924401]

[9] Bommareddy K, Hamade H, Lopez-Olivo MA, Wehner M, Tosh T, Barbieri JS. Association of spironolactone use with risk of cancer: A systematic review and meta-analysis. JAMA Dermatol 2022; 158(3): 275-82.
[http://dx.doi.org/10.1001/jamadermatol.2021.5866] [PMID: 35138351]

[10] Kelly Y, Tosti A. Androgenetic Alopecias: Clinical Treatments.Asz-Sigall D, Pirmes R Hair and Scalp Treatments. 1st ed. Switzerland: Springer 2020; pp. 91-108.
[http://dx.doi.org/10.1007/978-3-030-21555-2_8]

[11] Jung JY, Yeon JH, Choi JW, *et al.* Effect of dutasteride 0.5 mg/d in men with androgenetic alopecia recalcitrant to finasteride. Int J Dermatol 2014; 53(11): 1351-7.
[http://dx.doi.org/10.1111/ijd.12060] [PMID: 24898559]

[12] Hazlehurst JM, Oprescu AI, Nikolaou N, *et al.* Dual-5α-reductase inhibition promotes hepatic lipid accumulation in man. J Clin Endocrinol Metab 2016; 101(1): 103-13.
[http://dx.doi.org/10.1210/jc.2015-2928] [PMID: 26574953]

[13]   Traish AM. Health risks associated with long-term finasteride and dutasteride use: It's time to sound the alarm. World J Mens Health 2020; 38(3): 323-37.
[http://dx.doi.org/10.5534/wjmh.200012] [PMID: 32202088]

CHAPTER 51

Telogen Effluvium: Tips

Mohammad Reza Namazi[1],*

[1] *Shiraz University of Medical Sciences and Dr. Namazi Skin and Hair Clinic, Shiraz, Iran*

Telogen Effluvium (TE) is one of the most common causes of hair loss. Its causes are numerous and include illness, stress, nutritional deficiencies, drugs, thyroid diseases, scalp inflammation, changing time zone, over-the-counter drugs for weight loss, some herbal remedies, dieting, heavy exercise, esp. aerobic which causes more oxidative stress, *etc.* Many anti-hair loss and multi-vitamin supplements contain vitamin A and selenium which can cause hair loss at high serum levels [1].

Some other important tips on TE are provided:

- As 50% of the hair need to be lost for the scalp to become visible, thining is usually not a feature of TE, being especially unobvious to the physician. Rather, fullness of a patient's hairbrush with hair is typical. Bitemporal thinning, no change in hair diameter and decrease in ponytail length and thickness are found only in TE [1].

- The new method of hair pull test is suggested as follows:

It is possible to wash and brush at any time prior to the test. Around 50-60 hairs (a 4-6 mm bundle of hair depending upon the hair diameter) at the vertex are separated. The size of the bundle is based on experience and estimation. The bundle is held near the root and firmly pulled using slow traction as the fingers slide along the hair shaft. The force should suffice to mildly pull the scalp, making a slight uneasiness unassociated with pain. Broken hair is not counted; > 2 hairs is considered positive. When the test shows positivity in multiple scalp regions, telogen or anagen effluvium are taken into account. In the case of other hair disorders like alopecia areata, only the affected area will show a positive result. For the purpose of tracking the progression of alopecia areata, acute instances of telogen effluvium, anagen effluvium, and loose anagen syndrome, the hair pull test is most beneficially employed. The hair pull test proves to be most

---

*** Corresponding author Mohammad Reza Namazi:** Shiraz University of Medical Sciences and Dr. Namazi Skin and Hair Clinic, Shiraz, Iran; E-mail: rezanamazi12@yahoo.com

successful during the acute phases of severe conditions. Due to its low sensitivity and high interobserver variability, hair pull test is not recommended for use when dealing with patients who have a more chronic condition such as chronic telogen effluvium [2].

- In TE, CBC, TFT, ferritin and iron, zinc, B12, folate, vitamin A, and ANA (based on the presence of other symptoms) are requested. Biopsy is needed if definitive diagnosis is unclear [1]. Vitamin C increases iron absorption and its intake with iron is important for treating iron deficiency [3]. After stopping the trigger, hair shedding cessation and noticeable re-growth can take 3-6 months each, with significant cosmetic change possibly taking up to 12-18 months to appear [1].

- Topical and low dose (0.25-1.25 mg/d) oral minoxidil and topical steroids are effective. A short treatment with one injection of triamcinolone 40 mg per month in severe cases is suggested [1].

REFERENCES

[1]   Burroway B, Griggs J, Martinez-Velasco MA, Tosti A. Telogen effluvium. In: Tosti A, Ed. Asz-Sigall D, Pirmes R Hair and Scalp Treatments. 1st ed. Switzerland: Springer 2020; pp. 125-38.
       [http://dx.doi.org/10.1007/978-3-030-21555-2_10]

[2]   McDonald KA, Shelley AJ, Colantonio S, Beecker J. Hair pull test: Evidence-based update and revision of guidelines. J Am Acad Dermatol 2017; 76(3): 472-7.
       [http://dx.doi.org/10.1016/j.jaad.2016.10.002] [PMID: 28010890]

[3]   Almohanna HM. Ahmed AA, Tosti A. Role of oral supplements: When and How to choose. In: Tosti A, Ed. Asz-Sigall D, Pirmes R Hair and Scalp Treatments. 1st ed. Switzerland: Springer 2020; pp. 77-90.
       [http://dx.doi.org/10.1007/978-3-030-21555-2_7]

CHAPTER 52

Frontal Fibrosing Alopecia/lichen Planopilaris: Some Pearls

Mohammad Reza Namazi[1,*]

[1] *Shiraz University of Medical Sciences and Dr. Namazi Skin and Hair Clinic, Shiraz, Iran*

Frontal fibrosing alopecia is a patterned scarring hair loss along the frontal hair line, which is considered as a variant of lichen planopilaris by some experts.

-Finasteride 2.5-5 mg/d is considered the first line agent, with hydroxychlorouine and retinoids as the the second line agents [1]. Hydroxychloroquine dose can be increased up to 5 mg/kg/d. Its effect starts after 3-6 months. Higher doses for the first 6 weeks have accelerated the clinical response in rheumatoid arthritis [2], but are associated with an increased the risk of retinopathy. Smoking, and possibly proton pump inhibitors [3], may reduce its effect. Responsive cases should receive treatment for 2 years [1]. Hyperpigmentation is a side effect of hydroxychloroquine (Fig. **1**) which may be associated with bruising. Upon cessation of hydroxychloroquine, some patients demonstrate partial improvement, and laser treatments may improve the residual dyschromia [4].

Jak-inhibitors may be considered for resistant or rapidly progressive cases [5].

-Some resistant cases do not experience a remission with orally administered agents plus intralesional triamcinolone injections. In this situation, this author has used 5-FU-triamcinolone combination, a potent immunosuppressive and anti-fibrotic mixture, successfully. The maximum dose of 5-FU is 100 mg per session.

-As vitamin D deficiency is implicated in both autoimmunity and excessive scar formation, checking vitamin D levels is suggested.

- Facial papules reflecting the lichenoid inflammation of facial vellus hair follicles can occur in the backgrounds of frontal fibrosing alopecia, lichen planopilaris (LPP), or even alone (Fig. **2**). Isotretinoin (5-30 mg/d) is effective against them.

* **Corresponding author Mohammad Reza Namazi:** Shiraz University of Medical Sciences and Dr. Namazi Skin and Hair Clinic, Shiraz, Iran; E-mail: rezanamazi12@yahoo.com

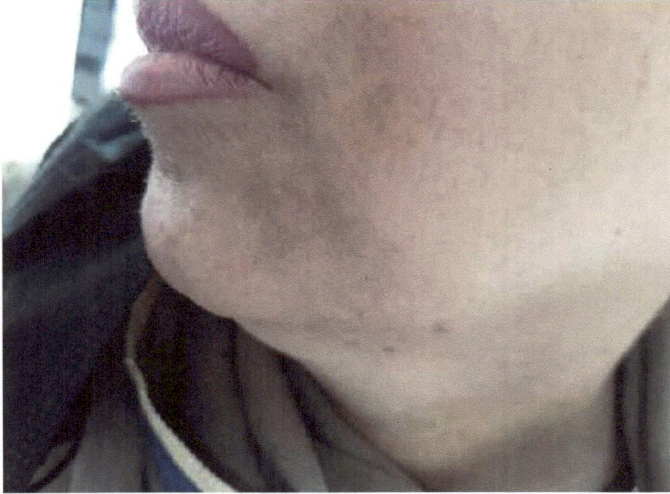

Fig. (1). Hydroxychloroquine-induced pigmentation on the marionette line and lateral chin.

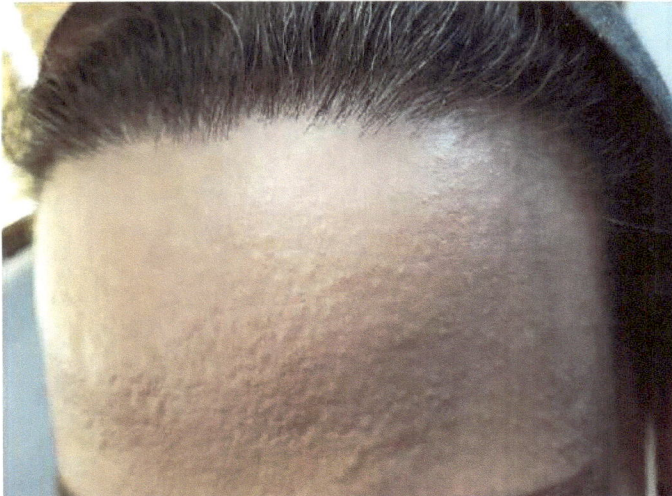

Fig. (2). Facial papules of lichen planopilaris associated with frontal fibrosing alopecia causing recession of the hair line.

-Lichen planopilaris of the scalp/beard/brow can present as a moderately progressive, irreversible, scarring alopecia and needs serious treatment with potent immunosuppressives ± intralesional injections. Using just topical steroids or calcineurin inhibitors can be an irremediable mistake. Regrowth may occur in early stages [1].

-This author had a very resistant case of lichen planopilaris unresponse to multiple treatments including finasteride 5 mg/d + hydroxychloroquine 200 mg/d + isotretinoin 40 mg/wk, intralesional 5-FU + triamcinolone, and baricitinib 4 mg/d who experienced complete remission with baricitinib 4 mg/d + isotretinoin 10 mg/d.

REFERENCES

[1]   Vano-Galvan S, Saceda-Corralo D, Pirmez R. Scarring alopecias. In: Tosti A, Ed. Asz-Sigall D, Pirmes R Hair and Scalp Treatments. 1st ed. Switzerland: Springer 2020; pp. 139-60.
[http://dx.doi.org/10.1007/978-3-030-21555-2_11]

[2]   Kalia S, Dutz JP. New concepts in antimalarial use and mode of action in dermatology. Dermatol Ther 2007; 20(4): 160-74.
[http://dx.doi.org/10.1111/j.1529-8019.2007.00131.x] [PMID: 17970883]

[3]   Namazi MR. The potential negative impact of proton pump inhibitors on the immunopharmacologic effects of chloroquine and hydroxychloroquine. Lupus 2009; 18(2): 104-5.
[http://dx.doi.org/10.1177/0961203308097574] [PMID: 19151110]

[4]   Bajoghli A, Hernandez G, Cardis MA. Hydroxychloroquine-induced Hyperpigmentation. J Rheumatol 2020; 47(11): 1721-2.
[http://dx.doi.org/10.3899/jrheum.200138] [PMID: 33139523]

[5]   Yang CC, Khanna T, Sallee B, Christiano AM, Bordone LA. Tofacitinib for the treatment of lichen planopilaris: A case series. Dermatol Ther 2018; 31(6): 12656.
[http://dx.doi.org/10.1111/dth.12656] [PMID: 30264512]

CHAPTER 53

Methotrexate Pearls

Mohammad Reza Namazi[1,*]

[1] Shiraz University of Medical Sciences and Dr. Namazi Skin and Hair Clinic, Shiraz, Iran

Methotrexate (MTX) is a medication used in low doses to treat inflammatory skin conditions and in much higher doses as a chemotherapy agent for leukemia and some cancers.

-Weekly doses of MTX vary from 5 to 30 mg. MTX is administered as a single dose weekly. Some clinicians divide the dose into three equal parts spaced 12 hours apart. It is suggested to prescribe folic acid in 1 mg/d for weekly doses of less than 15 mg, and in 5 mg/d for higher doses of MTX. Some suggest avoiding taking folic acid on the day(s) MTX is taken. Folic acid decreases mucositis, bone marrow and hepatic toxicities, and nausea [1].

-Consider test dose of 2.5–5 mg × 1 with F/U CBC and LFTs in 1 week. Then you can go directly to 15 mg/week [2].

-Elderly with little muscle mass may have serum BUN and creatinine in the normal range despite reduced glomerular filtration rate (GFR). Therefore, Cockcroft-Gault equation should be used to approximate GFR. If GFR is higher than 50 mL/min, no adjustment is needed. GFR of 10-50 mL/min stipulates dose reduction by 50% plus monitoring for toxicity and worsening renal function. GFR less than 10 mL/min is a contraindication to the use of MTX [1].

- MTX does not need to be discontinued for any surgery [3].

-In the author's experience, for those experiencing nausea with intramuscular injections, subcutaneous injections into the abdomen can be chosen as the drug is less rapidly absorbed from fatty tissues than muscles, causing fewer and less severe side effects.

Corresponding author Mohammad Reza Namazi: Shiraz University of Medical Sciences and Dr. Namazi Skin and Hair Clinic, Shiraz, Iran; E-mail: rezanamazi12@yahoo.com

REFERENCES

[1]   Bangert CA, Costner MI. Methotrexate in dermatology. Dermatol Ther 2007; 20(4): 216-28.
[http://dx.doi.org/10.1111/j.1529-8019.2007.00135.x] [PMID: 17970887]

[2]   Hylwa S, Hirliman E, Liu J, Luxenberg E, Boul C. Pocket Dermatology. 1st ed. Switzerland: Springer 2021; p. 407.
[http://dx.doi.org/10.1007/978-3-030-83602-3]

[3]   Dermnet. Methotrexate. Available from: https://dermnetnz.org/topics/methotrexate (Accessed 9/26/2022).

CHAPTER 54

Intravenous Immunoglobulin Pearls

Mohammad Reza Namazi[1,*]

[1] *Shiraz University of Medical Sciences and Dr. Namazi Skin and Hair Clinic, Shiraz, Iran*

Intravenous immunoglobulin (IVIG) is generally a safe and well-tolerated therapeutic modality.

-A total dose of 1–2 g/kg is administered over 3-5 days. Infusion is done slowly over 4–4.5 h.

-The fluid overload may not be tolerated by patients suffering from renal failure/congestive heart failure.

-Following the administration of IVIG, patients typically experience mild and short-lived symptoms such as flu-like symptoms, headache (most common), flushing, malaise, fever, chills, chest tightness, tiredness, myalgia, shortness of breath, back pain, nausea, vomiting, diarrhea, blood pressure changes, and increased heart rate, which are usually seen within the first 30 min of infusion. Consider slowing the infusion rate or temporary discontinuation. These reactions can be prevented by pre-medication with antihistamines, NSAIDs, and steroids.

-Anaphylaxis is rare and most probably occurs in IgA deficient patients.

-As a blood product, IVIG has the potential risk of transmission of viral infections.

-Aseptic meningitis is seen in less than 11% of patients (severe acute headache with neck rigidity, photophobia, fever, lethargy, nausea/vomiting) and usually recovers without complications [1].

-Thromboembolic problems (stroke/MI) are encountered with higher doses/higher infusion rates (because of hyperviscosity). Lyophilized IVIG products are implicated in over 70% of thrombotic complications. Patients who developed stroke had important risk factors like previous stroke, TIA, carotid artery stenosis,

* **Corresponding author Mohammad Reza Namazi:** Shiraz University of Medical Sciences and Dr. Namazi Skin and Hair Clinic, Shiraz, Iran; E-mail: rezanamazi12@yahoo.com

chronic hypertension, arrhythmia and hypercoagulable states. Cases who developed myocardial infarction had important risk factors such as previous myocardial infarction, hypertension, recent CABG, and diabetes. Risk factors for hyperviscosity such as low cardiac output, vascular problems, and high cholesterol levels should be enquired [2].

-Age $\geq$ 65, nephrotoxic drugs, diabetes, pre-existing renal disease, hypovolemia, and sepsis are reported to pre-dispose patients to renal toxicity with sucrose-containing IVIG. Patients having rheumatoid factor or cryoglobulin have an elevated risk of acute kidney failure and some recommend checking these factors prior to starting IVIG. The intake of renin-angiotensin system inhibitors is an important independent risk factor for acute renal failure [3].

-High-risk cases for kidney failure, thromboembolic problems, and aseptic meningitis should be hydrated.

-Patients with blood types A, B, or AB should be monitored with a hemoglobin workup two days after the therapy for hemolytic reaction as IVIG may contain anti- A or anti-B blood group antibodies [4].

-Of note, IVIG is used for treating sepsis and septic shock – another advantage in patients with both toxic epidermal necrolysis and septicemia [5].

-IVIG is safe to use in pregnancy and has even been used to improve the outcome in women with immune disorders [6].

REFERENCES

[1]   Hylwa S, Hirliman E, Liu J, Luxenberg E, Boul C. Pocket Dermatology. 1st ed. Switzerland: Springer 2021; pp. 435-8.
        [http://dx.doi.org/10.1007/978-3-030-83602-3]

[2]   Fernandez AP, Kerdel FA. The use of i.v. IG therapy in dermatology. Dermatol Ther 2007; 20(4): 288-305.
        [http://dx.doi.org/10.1111/j.1529-8019.2007.00142.x] [PMID: 17970894]

[3]   Moulis G, Sailler L, Sommet A, Lapeyre-Mestre M, Montastruc JL. Exposure to inhibitors of the renin–angiotensin system is a major independent risk factor for acute renal failure induced by sucrose-containing intravenous immunoglobulins: A case–control study. Pharmacoepidemiol Drug Saf 2012; 21(3): 314-9.
        [http://dx.doi.org/10.1002/pds.2253] [PMID: 21953992]

[4]   Arumugham VB, Rayi A. Intravenous immunoglobulin. Treasure Island: StatPearls Publishing 2022.

[5]   Alejandria MM, Lansang MAD, Dans LF, Mantaring JB III. Intravenous immunoglobulin for treating sepsis, severe sepsis and septic shock. Cochrane Libr 2013; 2018(12): CD001090.
        [http://dx.doi.org/10.1002/14651858.CD001090.pub2] [PMID: 24043371]

[6]   Habets DHJ, Pelzner K, Wieten L, Spaanderman MEA, Villamor E, Al-Nasiry S. Intravenous immunoglobulins improve live birth rate among women with underlying immune conditions and recurrent pregnancy loss: a systematic review and meta-analysis. Allergy Asthma Clin Immunol. 2022 Mar 11;18(1):23.
[http://dx.doi.org/10.1186/s13223-022-00660-8] [PMID: 35277202]

CHAPTER 55

A Simple, Limited Patch Testing

Mohammad Reza Namazi[1,*]

[1] *Shiraz University of Medical Sciences and Dr. Namazi Skin and Hair Clinic, Shiraz, Iran*

Humans are like fish living in an ocean full of allergens. A dermatologist who does not know contact dermatitis well cannot be considered a good general dermatologist. Patch testing is done for the investigation of the substances that have caused allergic contact dermatitis. Below, a simple patch testing is described:

-If you are very suspicious to an agent for causing allergic contact dermatitis, esp. when a formal patch testing is not possible or difficult for any reason, you can ask the patient to put the suspicious agent on his upper arm and cover it with a piece of cellophane fixed to the skin with a tape. It is kept for 48 hours, then the area is looked for any reactions. It can take up to 5 days for allergic reactions to form, so reading at 5 days is more definitive. Moreover, irritant reactions visible on earlier days should have diminished/disappeared by day 5.

-For latex gloves and fabrics, it is advisable to put a piece of the agent in hot water for a while and then put it on the arm - this increases the release of the allergen.

-Materials intended to be left on the skin, such as medicaments and cosmetics, are tested 'as is'; 'rinse-off' products, such as rinse-off cleansers, are tested at 5% dilution, and soaps, shampoos and detergents at 1% or less [1]. For making a 1% dilution of a shampoo, add 4.5 cc water to 0.5 cc of it and stir the mixture. Then, aspirate 0.05 cc of the mixture in a 0.5 cc syringe and fill the syringe with water.

-Prednisone >10 mg/d (10 mg/d is OK, but better if stopped for 3–5 days), cyclosporine >2 mg/kg/d, IM triamcinolone within the last 4 weeks, and topical steroid use on the testing site in the previous 3-7 days can lead to false negative patch testing [2].

* **Corresponding author Mohammad Reza Namazi:** Shiraz University of Medical Sciences and Dr. Namazi Skin and Hair Clinic, Shiraz, Iran; E-mail: rezanamazi12@yahoo.com

-For women having perioral hypermelanosis, consider post-inflammatory hyperpigmentation secondary to a subtle contact dermatitis to lipsticks, and proceed with patch-testing. Other causes include lip licker dermatitis and, in this author's experience, hyperpigmentation can occur secondary to a very subtle, chronic inflammation caused by xerosis of the peri-oral skin which seems to be more common in females.

-Isolated scalp itch may be caused by a very mild contact dermatitis to shampoos. Consider patch testing. Sodium lauryl sulphate-free shampoos may resolve the problem.

-Some patients with axillary contact dermatitis to perfume sprays deny applying them on the axillae. Do not get fooled by their negative response. They spray the perfumes on on the part of their clothes covering the axillary areas, not directly on the axillary skin!

-Metallic mobile phones may be the cause of unilateral ear contact dermatitis to nickel.

-Fingertip dermatitis may be caused by allergy to prayer beads used by Muslims.

REFERENCES

[1]   Willkinson SM, Beck MH. Contact dermatitis: Allergic. In: Burns T, Breathnach S, Cox N, Griffiths C, Eds. Rook's Textbook of Dermatology. 8th ed. Singapore: Wiley-Blackwell 2010; p. 2686.
[http://dx.doi.org/10.1002/9781444317633.ch25]

[2]   Hylwa S, Hirliman E, Liu J, Luxenberg E, Boul C. Pocket Dermatology. 1st ed. Switzerland: Springer 2021; pp. 380-1.
[http://dx.doi.org/10.1007/978-3-030-83602-3]

CHAPTER 56

Wet Wrap

Mohammad Reza Namazi[1,*]

[1] Shiraz University of Medical Sciences and Dr. Namazi Skin and Hair Clinic, Shiraz, Iran

Wet wrap is a very effective topical therapy for generalized dermatitis and other severe dermatoses like erythrodermic psoriasis. Do not take it lightly at all!

-Wet wrap is especially useful when a systemic immunosuppressive cannot be used, e.g because of a systemic infection, or when rapid control of a serious condition is aimed by adding wet wrap to a systemic immunosuppressive agent [1, 2]. Wet wrap is performed as follows:

• An emollient and/or steroid ointment is liberally applied to the area (usually an emollient is applied first and then a steroid ointment is applied on top of it).

• A tubular bandage or a bed linen soaked in warm water is wrapped on the area.

• The wet bandage/linen is covered with dry bandages or bed linens placed on top.

In case the chilly feeling becomes unpleasant, it is recommended to utilize two layers of dry wraps.

• A thick blanket is put on the patient, otherwise the patient may feel chilling.

• After 2-3 hours, the bandages/linens are removed (the patient may sleep on them overnight). The patient can take a shower and then put his dress on.

- In general, wet wrap is utilized for a few days until the inflammation has subsided. Emollients should be frequently applied throughout the day to maintain the desired outcomes in dermatitis.

---

* **Corresponding author Mohammad Reza Namazi:** Shiraz University of Medical Sciences and Dr. Namazi Skin and Hair Clinic, Shiraz, Iran; E-mail: rezanamazi12@yahoo.com

Wet wrap works via four diverse mechanisms:

• Cooling – The evaporation of water from the bandages aids in cooling the skin and reducing inflammation, itchiness, and soreness.

• Increased moisturizing – Wet bandages help facilitate the absorption of emollients into the skin, resulting in an extended moisturizing effect.

• Increased steroid penetration due to occlusion.

• The bandages protect the skin from the itching/scratching cycle, giving a chance to it to heal properly.

REFERENCES

[1]   Navrotski BRF, Nihi FM, Camilleri MJ, Cerci FB. Wet wrap dressings as a rescue therapy option for erythrodermic psoriasis. An Bras Dermatol 2018; 93(4): 598-600.
        [http://dx.doi.org/10.1590/abd1806-4841.20186414] [PMID: 30066777]

[2]   Dermnet. Wet Wrap. Available from: https://dermnetnz.org/topics/wet-wraps (Accessed 8/23/2022).

CHAPTER 57

Management of Varicose Veins

Mohammad Reza Namazi[1,*]

[1] Shiraz University of Medical Sciences and Dr. Namazi Skin and Hair Clinic, Shiraz, Iran

Chronic venous disorders span from spider veins, reticular veins, and varicose veins to chronic venous insufficiency, which may involve edema, hyperpigmentation, and venous ulcers.

-In upright position, 0.1 mm < veins < 1 mm are telangiectasia, 1 mm ≤ veins < 3 mm are reticular veins and veins ≥ 3 mm are varicose veins.

-Varicosities may occur secondary to genetic proneness, valvular incompetence, weakening of vascular walls, and elevated intravenous pressure. Prolonged standing; enhanced intra-abdominal pressure due to obesity, pregnancy and chronic constipation; deep venous thrombosis causing valvular damage; pelvic tumors or metastasis to groin lymph nodes; and arteriovenous fistula secondary to surgery or war injury may be contributing factors.

-While varicose veins can result in different levels of discomfort or cosmetic problems, they rarely lead to significant complications. Indications of a more severe underlying vascular insufficiency can manifest as alterations in skin coloration, dermatitis, superficial thrombophlebitis, venous ulcer formation, and lipodermatosclerosis.

-Varicose veins can cause pain, itching and burning sensations. Pain caused by varicosities is increased with prolonged standing, being worse in the afternoon and night. The patients may put pillows under their legs at night or massage the legs to decrease pain. In contrast, pain caused by ischemia is alleviated by suspending the legs and exacerbated by elevating them. Ischemic pain exacerbates but varicose pain usually improves with walking.

-Fan-shaped, abnormally visible vessels at the ankle (corona phlebectatica) are early indicators of advanced venous insufficiency Fig. (**1**). Diminished ankle mo-

---

* **Corresponding author Mohammad Reza Namazi:** Shiraz University of Medical Sciences and Dr. Namazi Skin and Hair Clinic, Shiraz, Iran; E-mail: rezanamazi12@yahoo.com

bility, atrophie blanche, and lipodermatosclerosis also indicate an advanced venous disorder.

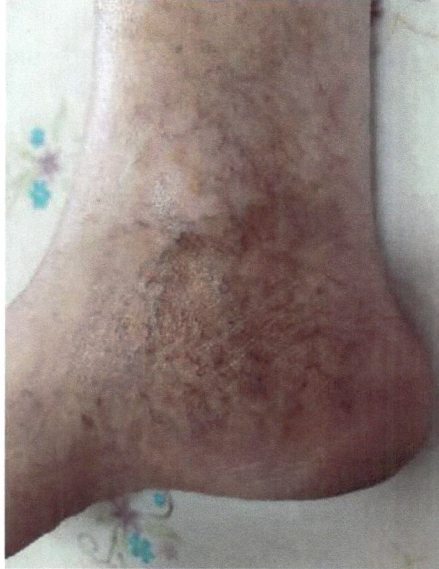

Fig. (1). Fan-shaped, abnormally visible vessels at the ankle, called corona phlebectasia, is an early pointer to advanced venous insufficiency.

-In cases of severe venous disease or when considering interventional therapy, venous duplex ultrasonography emerges as the most favored modality (from both pelvic and leg veins). Sonography should be performed in both recumbent and standing positions, while performing the Valsalva maneuver or compressing the leg.

-Interventional treatments include thermal ablation (external laser for telangiectasias and endovenous laser or radio waves for larger veins), sclerotherapy, and surgery. A mounting body of literature does not consistently endorse surgery as the preferred interventional treatment method. Surgery is considered as the third-line option after sclerotheraspy and endovenous thermal ablation [1].

-Conservative treatment options are considered for cases who are excluded from interventional treatments or do not consent to them or are pregnant. These measures include external compression; lifestyle changes, such as refraining from lengthy standing and straining, exercise, and sporting loose-fitting garments, Modifying cardiovascular risk factors; alleviating peripheral edema; elevating the affected leg; losing weight; and phlebotonics.

-The first line of treatment for varicose veins has traditionally been compression therapy. However, it is unclear if compression stockings effectively treat varicose veins unassociated with active or healed venous ulcers. External compression is considered only if interventional treatment is ineffectual or as the initial treatment just in pregnancy [1]. If compression stockings are used, class II is used for varicosities and class I for reticular veins. Class II exerts more pressure. Stocking is worn from above the toes to below the knee. The patient should remove it at night to prevent pressure ulcers. Distal pulse should be checked prior to recommending compression stockings. If the patient has ischemic ulcer as well, compression exacerbates it and should not be used. If there is bilateral edema, compression cannot be used unless heart failure is ruled out. Obese patients for whom an appropriate size stocking may be unavailable and the elderly who may have difficulty wearing stockings can use elastic bandage instead. Elastic bandage should be worn in a way that it is tighter distally and looser proximally.

-Phlebotonics, such as flavonoids, grape seed extract, horse chestnut seed extract, *etc.* may decrease symptoms of chronic venous insufficiency and are available as multiple agents in one supplement [1]. Based on high quality evidence, Daflon (micronized purified flavonoid fraction) is effective in alleviating leg symptoms, edema and quality of life in individuals with chronic venous disorder [2]. Multiple randomised controlled studies have shown the efficacy of Daflon 500 mg in venous leg ulcers [3]. As a side-note, Daflon can be helpful in the management of lymphatic disorders as well, as biofalvonoids stimulate the generation of new capillary lymphatic networks which cause an increase in lymph re-absorption [4].

-Pentoxifylline can help venous ulcers heal more quickly. A larger dose, *i.e.* 800 mg thrice daily, is more effective than smaller doses [5]. Combination therapy with hydroxychloroquine may reduce the symptoms more effectively [6].

-Ultrasound therapy may offer the relief of erythema, hardness and pain [7].

-Sildenafil, a phosphodiesterase (PDE) 5 inhibitor used for erectile dysfunction, exerts anti-inflammtory, anti-platelet aggregation, anti-fibrosis, and vasodilatory effects. It improves the endothelial dysfunction in preeclampsia and the healing of wounds in scleroderma and diabetes [8]. Its effect on venous ulcers warrants clinical studies.

REFERENCES

[1]   Raetz J, Wilson M, Collins K. Varicose veins: Diagnosis and treatment. Am Fam Physician 2019; 99(11): 682-8.
       [PMID: 31150188]

[2]   Kakkos SK, Nicolaides AN. Efficacy of micronized purified flavonoid fraction (Daflon®) on improving individual symptoms, signs and quality of life in patients with chronic venous disease: A

systematic review and meta-analysis of randomized double-blind placebo-controlled trials. Int Angiol 2018; 37(2): 143-54.
[http://dx.doi.org/10.23736/S0392-9590.18.03975-5] [PMID: 29385792]

[3]   Katsenis K. Micronized purified flavonoid fraction (MPFF): A review of its pharmacological effects, therapeutic efficacy and benefits in the management of chronic venous insufficiency. Curr Vasc Pharmacol 2005; 3(1): 1-9.
[http://dx.doi.org/10.2174/1570161052773870] [PMID: 15641940]

[4]   Shishlo VK, Malinin AA, Diufzhanov AA. [Mechanisms of antioedemic effect of bioflavonoids in experiment]. Angiol Sosud Khir 2013; 19(2): 25-30.
[PMID: 23863788]

[5]   Falanga V, Fujitani RM, Diaz C, *et al.* Systemic treatment of venous leg ulcers with high doses of pentoxifylline: efficacy in a randomized, placebo-controlled trial. Wound Repair Regen 1999; 7(4): 208-13.
[http://dx.doi.org/10.1046/j.1524-475X.1999.00208.x] [PMID: 10781212]

[6]   Choonhakarn C, Chaowattanapanit S. Lipodermatosclerosis: Improvement noted with hydroxychloroquine and pentoxifylline. J Am Acad Dermatol 2012; 66(6): 1013-4.
[http://dx.doi.org/10.1016/j.jaad.2011.11.942] [PMID: 22583718]

[7]   Damian DL, Yiasemides E, Gupta S, Armour K. Ultrasound therapy for lipodermatosclerosis. Arch Dermatol 2009; 145(3): 330-2.
[http://dx.doi.org/10.1001/archdermatol.2009.24] [PMID: 19289773]

[8]   Kniotek M, Boguska A. Sildenafil can affect innate and adaptive immune system in both experimental animals and patients. J Immunol Res 2017; 2017: 1-8.
[http://dx.doi.org/10.1155/2017/4541958] [PMID: 28316997]

CHAPTER 58

Improving Scar Formation: Pearls

Mohammad Reza Namazi[1,*]

[1] *Shiraz University of Medical Sciences and Dr. Namazi Skin and Hair Clinic, Shiraz, Iran*

Scar formation is a big concern for both patients and physicians. Below, some important points in this regard are mentioned:

-Amazingly, fetal wounds, esp. in the first 6 months of gestation, heal without scar formation. Fetal skin contains more hyaluronic acid, which attracts more water molecules, hence fetal tissues are more fluid and facilitate cellular movement. Fetal wounds have fewer pro-inflammatory cytokines that downregulate hyaluronic acid expression.

-*In vivo* experiments indicate that tamoxifen delays wound healing but improves scar formation by decreasing TGF-β1 which stimulates the synthesis of collagen and scar formation. This may be applicable to a wide range of conditions characterized by excess collagen deposition and scar formation like keloids, burns, recipient site necrosis in hair transplantation, neurofibromatosis, and epidermolysis bullosa [1].

-Losartan, an angiotensin II type 1 receptor antagonist, is an inhibitor of TGF-β1 and some reports have shown its efficacy in decreasing the scarring in dystrophic epidermolysis bullosa [2]. *In vivo* studies have also shown topical losartan to decrease scarring [3].

- Fenofibrate is shown to suppress TGF-β1/Smad3 signaling pathway and attenuate fibrosis in a rat model of diabetic nephropathy [4, 5] and also experimental pulmonary fibrosis [5, 6]. This interesting observation can be applicable to skin scarring conditions and awaits clinical trials.

-Interestingly, low dose topical steroids suppress hypergranulation, reduce exudate, and accelerate wound healing [7]. Low dose topical steroids may decrease scar formation through decreasing inflammation. Animal studies have

* **Corresponding author Mohammad Reza Namazi:** Shiraz University of Medical Sciences and Dr. Namazi Skin and Hair Clinic, Shiraz, Iran; E-mail: rezanamazi12@yahoo.com

shown that acute, high-dose systemic corticosteroids have no effect on wound healing, whereas chronic systemic steroids may cause impairment [8].

-Vitamin D decreases fibrosis [9], and vitamin D supplementation may provide some protection against keloids and fibrotic processes.

-There is no robust evidence that acceleration of healing with some agents such as Cicamosa, Cicalfate, Repair creams, or Biafine is associated with decreased scar formation. It should be noted that from a theoretical standpoint, promotion of fibroblast activation may induce more scarring. Moreover, in postmenopausal women, wounds heal slowly but leave less scarring [1]. Biafine emulsion is a good wound healing and anti-inflammatory agent which contains trolamine, a macrophage recruiter. Macrophagres expedite wound healing [10]. It can also be used for treating post-radiation acute dermatitis. Its possible effect in reducing scar formation via anti-inflammatory effects needs researching.

-Botulinum toxin directly suppresses fibroblast proliferation. Several reports have demonstrated its efficacy for prevention of hypertrophic scars and the reduction of pain and pruritus of keloids [11]. Intradermal injection of high dose Botox (8 U at each point, with an interval of 1 cm) from a site 5 mm away from the wound edge immediately after surgery has enhanced the cosmesis of the scars [12].

- Sildenafil, a phosphodiesterase (PDE) 5 inhibitor used for erectile dysfunction, improves fibrosis in scleroderma through increasing cyclic GMP levels in fibroblasts, resulting in the decrease of several pro-fibrotic factors that are upregulated by TGF-β1 [13]. Sildenafil may be effective in other scarring conditions like burns, epidermolysis bullosa, and even keloid proneness. It also possesses anti-inflammtory effects [14].

- A systematic review and meta-analysis has shown massaging burn scars can significantly improve scar formation and reduce pruritus and anxiety [15].

Vacuum massage is performed with a mechanical device that lifts the skin by means of suction. Currently, there is not ample evidence for the efficacy of this treatment; however, improvement of the tissue hardness and skin elasticity are reported. There is little information on the decrease of pain and itch due to vacuum massage. Vacuum massage may release the mechanical tension associated with scar retraction and thus induce apoptosis of myofibroblasts [16, 17].

REFERENCES

[1]   Namazi MR, Fallahzadeh MK, Schwartz RA. Strategies for prevention of scars: What can we learn from fetal skin? Int J Dermatol 2011; 50(1): 85-93.
[http://dx.doi.org/10.1111/j.1365-4632.2010.04678.x] [PMID: 21039435]

[2]   Pourani MR, Vahidnezhad H, Mansouri P, *et al.* Losartan treatment improves recessive dystrophic epidermolysis bullosa: A case series. Dermatol Ther 2022; 35(7): 15515.
[http://dx.doi.org/10.1111/dth.15515] [PMID: 35420725]

[3]   Zhao WY, Zhang LY, Wang ZC, *et al.* The compound losartan cream inhibits scar formation *via* TGF-β/Smad pathway. Sci Rep 2022; 12(1): 14327.
[http://dx.doi.org/10.1038/s41598-022-17686-y] [PMID: 35995975]

[4]   Al-Rasheed NM, Al-Rasheed NM, Al-Amin MA, *et al.* Fenofibrate attenuates diabetic nephropathy in experimental diabetic rat's model *via* suppression of augmented TGF- β 1/Smad3 signaling pathway. Arch Physiol Biochem 2016; 122(4): 186-94.
[http://dx.doi.org/10.3109/13813455.2016.1164186] [PMID: 26959841]

[5]   Namazi MR, Parvizi MM. Fenofibrates: A safe and novel weapon against coronavirus-induced lung fibrosis. Int J Prev Med 2022; 13(1): 145.
[PMID: 37081857]

[6]   Kikuchi R, Maeda Y, Tsuji T, *et al.* Fenofibrate inhibits TGF-β-induced myofibroblast differentiation and activation in human lung fibroblasts *in vitro.* FEBS Open Bio 2021; 11(8): 2340-9.
[http://dx.doi.org/10.1002/2211-5463.13247] [PMID: 34228906]

[7]   Guo S, DiPietro LA. Factors affecting wound healing. J Dent Res 2010; 89(3): 219-29.
[http://dx.doi.org/10.1177/0022034509359125] [PMID: 20139336]

[8]   Wang AS, Armstrong EJ, Armstrong AW. Corticosteroids and wound healing: Clinical considerations in the perioperative period. Am J Surg 2013; 206(3): 410-7.
[http://dx.doi.org/10.1016/j.amjsurg.2012.11.018] [PMID: 23759697]

[9]   Mamdouh M, Omar GA, Hafiz HSA, Ali SM. Role of vitamin D in treatment of keloid. J Cosmet Dermatol 2022; 21(1): 331-6.
[http://dx.doi.org/10.1111/jocd.14070] [PMID: 33721390]

[10]   Cohen JL, Jorizzo JL, Kircik LH. Use of a topical emulsion for wound healing. J Support Oncol 2007; 5(10): 1-9.
[PMID: 18338743]

[11]   Alster TS, Harrison IS. Alternative clinical indications of botulinum toxin. Am J Clin Dermatol 2020; 21(6): 855-80.
[http://dx.doi.org/10.1007/s40257-020-00532-0] [PMID: 32651806]

[12]   Chen Z, Chen Z, Pang R, *et al.* The effect of botulinum toxin injection dose on the appearance of surgical scar. Sci Rep 2021; 11(1): 13670.
[http://dx.doi.org/10.1038/s41598-021-93203-x] [PMID: 34211099]

[13]   Higuchi T, Kawaguchi Y, Takagi K, *et al.* Sildenafil attenuates the fibrotic phenotype of skin fibroblasts in patients with systemic sclerosis. Clin Immunol 2015; 161(2): 333-8.
[http://dx.doi.org/10.1016/j.clim.2015.09.010] [PMID: 26387628]

[14]   Kniotek M, Boguska A. Sildenafil can affect innate and adaptive immune system in both experimental animals and patients. J Immunol Res 2017; 2017: 1-8.
[http://dx.doi.org/10.1155/2017/4541958] [PMID: 28316997]

[15]   Lin TR, Chou FH, Wang HH, Wang RH. Effects of scar massage on burn scars: A systematic review and meta-analysis. J Clin Nurs 2022.
[PMID: 35758338]

[16]   Moortgat P, Meirte J, Van Daele U, Anthonissen M, Vanhullebusch T, Maertens K. Vacuum massage in the treatment of scars. 2020 Dec 8. In: Téot L, Mustoe TA, Middelkoop E, Gauglitz GG, Eds. Textbook on Scar Management: State of the Art Management and Emerging Technologies. Cham, CH: Springer 2020.https://www.ncbi.nlm.nih.gov/books/NBK586069/ [Internet]

[17]   Moortgat P, Anthonissen M, Meirte J, Van Daele U, Maertens K. The physical and physiological effects of vacuum massage on the different skin layers: A current status of the literature. Burns Trauma 2016; 4: 41038-016-0053-9.
[http://dx.doi.org/10.1186/s41038-016-0053-9] [PMID: 27660766]

CHAPTER 59

Miscellaneous Medical Pearls

Mohammad Reza Namazi[1,*]

[1] Shiraz University of Medical Sciences and Dr. Namazi Skin and Hair Clinic, Shiraz, Iran

-Children are usually fearful of physicians and try to avoid physical examinations. They may think that their vaccinations were done because medical personnel/doctors did not like them and that this punishment may be repeated! A simple but remarkably calming sentence while trying to exam a child is: "What a nice child he (or she) is!". Saying this sentence makes children less tense and is far better than being silent.

-While prescribing topical creams or ointments for peri-anal dermatoses of children, tell the mother to just apply the topical and refrain from massaging the area with it. Massaging the peri-anal area in children can cause a pleasure feeling which might trigger a tendency toward receptive anal sex later in life.

-Do not get fooled by some rare patients who report the negative comment a colleague made about you or your procedure. Definitely, there may be some colleagues who may not observe ethical codes and try to backstab you. However, there are also some patients that for unknown reasons like to lie, to exaggerate a mildly negative comment, or to report a neutral comment as a negative one. I call this abnormal behavior as "Thais disease". Thais was the name of Alexander's mistress who enticed him into firing Persepolis. People having Thais disease may be rare, but they can provoke intense, impactful interpersonal conflicts. Be very careful while commenting about a colleague or his/her procedure, as the patient may be a case of "Thais disease".

-A very effective topical for thick plaques of psoriasis/sebopsoriasis of the scalp which do not responsd well to clobetasol lotion is 20% propylene glycol + 4-6% lactic acid in clobetasol lotion. The propylene glycol and lactic acid exert additive keratolytic effects, causing rapid resolution of the condition.

-For patients having corns/callosities on the sides of toes, esp. those having abnormal toes, wearing shoes made of textiles are advisable. Textile is softer and

---

* **Corresponding author Mohammad Reza Namazi:** Shiraz University of Medical Sciences and Dr. Namazi Skin and Hair Clinic, Shiraz, Iran; E-mail: rezanamazi12@yahoo.com

more moldable than leather and causes less pressure on the toes.

-Methotrexate is usually very effective against nail psoriasis. This author had a patient suffering from nail psoriasis who did not improve with adalimumab but showed a dramatic response to methotrexate. On the other hand, a patient with severe nail psoriais who did not respond to intramatricial triamcinolone and oral methotrexate responded partially to adalimumab.

-Actinic purpura may be, along with osteoporosis, a sign of collagen loss in skin and bone. The changes in skin collagen may correspond to changes in bone density [1]. Therefore, in patients with severe actinic purpuric lesions, fracture risk assessment may be warranted.

-Dapsone is usually very effective for disseminated granuloma annulare. For resistant cases, thalidomide can induce remission (J. Jorzo, personal communication, May 2008)[1].

-Thalidomide can be effective against resistant cases of pyoderma gangrenosum. (J. Jorzo, personal communication, May 2008).

-In this author's experience, cyclosporine is remarkably effective for prurigo nodularis of unknown cause, along with psychologic/psychiatric approaches if needed. It may be effective in resistant lichen simplex chronicus as well. Adding a potent topical anti-itch compound containing menthol, phenol and camphor, as mentioned in the previous chapters, can be of help. Cyclosporine is also usually effective in cases of resistant itch when no specific cause can be identified.

-I have not found n-acetylcysteine to be particularly effective against prurigo nodularis and lichen simplex chronicus, though some publications claim its efficacy.

-While encountering itch in renal failure patients, always check phosphate levels as elevated phosphate levels can cause itch. In this case, phosphate binding agents such as Renagel provide relief.

-Easy bruising can be caused by Ehlers-Danlos syndrome. Do not forget to evaluate patients for this syndrome whenever you face easy bruising.

-My experience with two cases of the very rare disorder delusional parasitosis is that risperidone cannot effectively control this disease, while pimozide can.

-The dose of TNF-alpha inhibitors in dissecting cellulitis of the scalp is the same as psoriasis, not as hidradenitis suppurativa.

-In my experience, intralesional 5-FU is effective for treatment of morphea plaques.

-Elephantiasis nostras verruciformis or lymphatic papillomatosis is a rare form of chronic lymphedema that causes progressive cutaneous hypertrophy. Topical calcipotriol can be of help in managing this condition.

-In my experience, dilute KOH (5-10%) in the treatment of molluscum contagiosum is not very effective and may leave superficial scars, esp. in children. Commercial products containing 10% salicylic acid and 0.5% fluorouracil, i.e. Verrumal and Actikerall solutions, are more tolerable, even in children, and also more efficacious. In small children, the application of topical anesthetic may be needed to prevent the burning sensation caused by the application of this compound. It can be applied every other day or less frequently.

Parents should be advised to refrain from using exfoliating washcloth for these children, as it can cause spreading of the lesions.

-While it is stated in most references that tretinoin is effective against flat verrucae, in my experience, there are lots of treatment failures and also intolerance due to skin irritation. Also, dilute KOH (5-10%), a keratolytic agent, is not a good choice as it may leave superficial scars, esp. in children. Cryotherapy and Verrumal or Actikerall solutions are better options.

-If you need to prescribe neotigason for a child who cannot take the capsule, the contents of the capsule can be suspended in arachis oil or olive oil (it is insoluble in water). An arbitrary 7 day expiry date is generally used for the mixture. Neotigasone is light sensitive and therefore it is important to prevent exposure of the capsule contents to light; further, the bottle in which the suspension is made should be of dark glass and covered in aluminium foil [2].

-Though some case reports have linked mycophenolate mofetil (MMF) to rising hepatitis C viral titres, its safety in patients with hepatitis B and C is documented [3].

-In my experience, Aven Cicalfate cream has good anti-inflammatory effect and can replace topical steroids for some situations like post-laser erythema.

-For managing hair loss, some physicians prescribe zinc supplements without checking serum zinc levels. However, zinc decreases the absorption of copper, causing copper deficiency.

-Facial burning and scalp itch may be manifestations of anxiety.

-White fabrics are preferable to dark ones for eczema patients, as the dyes are released from fabrics by sweating and can exacerbate the dermatitis. Yellow fabrics are also usually well tolerated.

-Perfumes used in make-ups can irritate sensitive skin. Almay Company produces hypo-allergenic makeups. Clinique products also usually have low amounts of perfumes.

-What to do if a patient gets runny eyes with a sunscreen? Chemical sunscreens can cause allergic contact reaction, which may appear only on the conjunctiva as it has no barrier to external agents. Changing the sunscreen to a physical one helps.

-Some patients with generalized hyperhidrosis respond well to oxybutynin 5 mg BD. Clonidine can also be effective in this condition.

-For hyperhidrosis of the axilla and even many cases of palmar and plantar hyperhidrosis, 20% aluminium chloride in absolute ethanol is remarkably effective. However, it can irritate the facial skin and eyes because of its alcoholic base. The following compound can be used for facial hyperhidrosis: 3 Amp. Atropin in Cold cream #30 gr.

-Applying topicals against the direction of the hair can cause traumatic folliculitis papules, which are finer than infectious folliculitis papules. This is also true regarding shaving.

-As zinc pyrithione has anti-bacterial (including anti-staph) activity [4], zinc pyrithione shampoo can be considered in the management of scalp folliculitis. Some physicians advise these patients to add betadine scrub to their shampoos. These patients usually respond well to doxycycline, which is effective against community acquired methicillin-resistant staph aureus (CA-MRSA). A dose of 200 mg/d is generally used for cutaneous CA-MRSA infections. The duration of therapy varies based on clinical response, with an average duration of treatment ranging from 10 to 21 days. Clindamycine, fluoroquinolones, rifampin, linezolid and daptomycine are other effective antibiotics against CA-MRSA [5]. The emergence of clindamycine resistant strains has limited the use of clindamycine for reating CA-MRSA [6]. Interestingly, when used in combination with rifampin, doxycycline may prevent the emergence of CA-MRSA strains resistant to rifampin. Importantly, unlike rifampin and fluoroquinolones, there is no evidence of rapid emergence of bacterial resistance when doxycycline is used as monotherapy to treat cutaneous CA-MRSA infections. For abscesses caused by CA-MRSA, incision and drainage is the single most important intervention [5]. This author has seen a case of tufted folliculitis, a condition with a possible pathogenic role of *S. aureus*, who did not respond to doxycyclin but was controlled with clindamycin-rifampin combination (both at 300 mg/d).

Gram-positive organisms are the dominant pathogens in skin and soft tissue infections, and MRSA comprises around 50% of *S. aureus* isolates. Accordingly, skin and soft tissue infections of a severity requiring hospitalization and antimicrobials should be treated with an agent effective against MRSA until susceptibility data are available. Covering gram-negative organisms may not be justifiable, esp. in immunocompetent patients. Gram-negatives, drug-resistant pathogens, and anaerobes are usually present in long-standing infection, particularly in the chronic diabetic foot infection [6].

-Smoking, excessive alcohol intake, emotional stress, physical illness and obesity are risk factors for canities [7].

-For patients having hand dermatitis caused/exacerbated by frequent washing, esp. those with dermatitis of the back of the hands, just sanitizing the palms and not the backs of the hands prior to eating, instead of washing by a soap, is usually better tolerated.

-Advise patients with intertrigo and groin problems not to wear jeans, plastic or woolen pants, and plastic underwear, esp. in summer.

-Some points on biologics [8]:

• Patients with latent T.B. should receive treatment for 2 weeks before the start of biologics.

• Biologics should be stopped for 6–12 months before live vaccines. Live vaccines should not be given to infants ≤ 6 months whose mothers have received biologics beyond 16 weeks' gestation.

• Certolizumab pegol is the biologic of choice for psoriasis in women planning conception. Consider stopping biologic therapy in the second/third trimester.

• If required, the dose of biologics or the interval of their use can be changed for a better response: Adalimumab can be used every week, Etanercept can be used twice weekly, Infliximab can be used every 6 weeks, Ustekinumab 45 mg every 12 weeks (≤100 kg) can be used as 90 mg every 8 or 12 weeks and Ustekinumab 90 mg every 12 weeks (> 100 kg) can be used as Ustekinumab 90 mg every 8 weeks (> 100 kg).

-For treating actinic keratosis, rather than using 5-FU 5% cream (Efudix), some experts use Actikerall or Verrumal solutions, which contain 0.5% 5-Fu and 10%

salicylic acid. Fluorouracil 0.5% may be safer, more tolerable, and as efficacious as fluorouracil 5% for managing actinic keratoses [9]. Compounding 0.5% 5-FU with 10% salicylic acid can dramatically increase its penetration, producing a faster response.

-Pyoderma gangrenosum can present as folliculitis or acneform lesions unresponsive to antibiotics.

This author had a patient with pyoderma gangrenosum taking mycophenolate mofetil for pulmonary lupus who did not respond to the addition of low dose cyclosporine. The patient could not take prednisolone because of severe osteoporosis. The addition of tacrolimus and tofacitinib, each separately, to mycophenolate and low dose cyclosporine, could not control the disease. The disease was well controlled with high dose cyclosporine.

REFERENCES

[1]   Shuster S. Osteoporosis, a unitary hypothesis of collagen loss in skin and bone. Med Hypotheses 2005; 65(3): 426-32.
[http://dx.doi.org/10.1016/j.mehy.2005.04.027] [PMID: 15951132]

[2]   Wakelin SH. Handbook of Systemic Drug Treatment in Dermatology. 1st ed. London: Manson Publishing Ltd 2002; p. 225.
[http://dx.doi.org/10.1201/b16367]

[3]   Zwerner J, Fiorentino D. Mycophenolate mofetil. Dermatol Ther 2007; 20(4): 229-38.
[http://dx.doi.org/10.1111/j.1529-8019.2007.00136.x] [PMID: 17970888]

[4]   Blanchard C, Brooks L, Ebsworth-Mojica K, *et al.* Zinc pyrithione improves the antibacterial activity of silver sulfadiazine ointment. MSphere 2016; 1(5): e00194-16.
[http://dx.doi.org/10.1128/mSphere.00194-16] [PMID: 27642637]

[5]   Bhambri S, Kim G. Use of oral doxycycline for community-acquired methicillin-resistant staphylococcus aureus (CA-MRSA) infections. J Clin Aesthet Dermatol 2009; 2(4): 45-50.
[PMID: 20729939]

[6]   Cardona AF, Wilson SE. Skin and soft-tissue infections: A critical review and the role of telavancin in their treatment. Clin Infect Dis 2015; 61: S69-78.
[http://dx.doi.org/10.1093/cid/civ528] [PMID: 26316560]

[7]   Tosti A, Ed. Most common patient hair questions. Asz-Sigall D, Pirmez R Hair and Scalp Treatments: A Practical Guide. 1st ed. Switzerland: Springer 2020; p. 325.

[8]   Jiyad Z, Flohr C. Handbook of Skin Disease Management. 1st ed. India: John Wiley & Sons Ltd. 2023; pp. 194-8.
[http://dx.doi.org/10.1002/9781119829072.app2]

[9]   Jorizzo JL, Carney PS, Ko WT, Robins P, Weinkle SH, Werschler WP. Fluorouracil 5% and 0.5% creams for the treatment of actinic keratosis: Equivalent efficacy with a lower concentration and more convenient dosing schedule. Cutis 2004; 74(6): 18-23.
[PMID: 15666898]

Publication Pearls

CHAPTER 60

Publication Pearls

Mohammad Reza Namazi[1,*]

[1] Shiraz University of Medical Sciences and Dr. Namazi Skin and Hair Clinic, Shiraz, Iran

"The purpose of research is to publish" - Michael Faraday, English Physicist and Chemist (1791–1867).

If you would like to step into the publication world, you should have the patience of Job, the longevity of Noah, and the faith of Abraham (faith in science). Do not get disappointed at all! I am exaggerating and just would like to increase your patience and tenaciousness. Publishing a paper may take a long time. You may face rejection from several journals, esp. if you would like to publish your paper in the highest impact factor journal as possible. In this case, you need to step down from the impact factor ladder until the highest impact factor journal possible accepts your work, which is time-consuming. Therefore, be very patient and tenacious. Memorize what Ferdowsi, a great Persian poet, has elegantly said regarding the utmost importance of papers:

"Our writings will remain, while we will go. Nothing will remain in the world from us, except our writings."

Below, some pearls and tricks for publishing papers will be given:

-If your research is unique in some aspects, it is important to mention this in the title and make your title eye-catching. For example, if you have done a research on the epidemiology of pemphigus in your area for the first time, mention it in the title, *e.g.* "Epidemiology of Pemphigus in Southern Iran: The first Study". If you have included a noticeably large number of cases or have used data gathered over many years, do mention that: " Epidemiology of Pemphigus in Southern Iran: a 20-year Retrospective Study" or "ABO Blood Groups and Pemphigus Vulgaris: A Study on 201 Patients".

*** Corresponding author Mohammad Reza Namazi:** Shiraz University of Medical Sciences and Dr. Namazi Skin and Hair Clinic, Shiraz, Iran; E-mail: rezanamazi12@yahoo.com

-If you have done a research on a disease prevalent in your area but you have not included many cases, especially if you have a negative result, which is not so desirable for editors to publish, you may have a higher chance of getting acceptance if you submit your paper to a journal the editor of which is from an area where that disease is rare or uncommon. For example, a negative result on the relationship between pemphigus vulgaris and ABO blood groups has more chance to get published in a Western journal than an Eastern one, as pemphigus is much less common in the West. An example is the following paper: Shahkar H, Fallahzadeh MK, Namazi MR. ABO blood groups and pemphigus vulgaris: No relationship. *Acta Dermatovenerol Alp Pannonica Adriat*. 2010;19(1):49-51. This paper is published in a western dermatology journal, but its publication in an Eastern journal would have been very difficult.

-For getting more citations, refrain from using uncommon words in the title of your paper; use the most common words. For example, if you chose "A Hypothesis on The Pathomechanism of Psoriasis" as the title, your work will get fewer citations than choosing "A Hypothesis on the Pathophysiology of Psoriasis". Researchers usually search the medical database with the most common words such as "Psoriasis and Pathophysiology" not with "Psoriasis and Pathomechanism". Another related point is that publishing in a journal indexed in PubMed is preferable to other journals which are not indexed in PubMed even if they are listed in Scopus or other important databases, as researchers definitely search Pubmed but may not search other databases. Also, note that for seeing the list of your publications, many people search only PubMed with your name.

-Throughout your paper, try to maximize your work. For example, one of my coworkers wrote the result section of our papers as: "Nine patients with fifteen scars were treated with emulsified fat…". I changed it to: "Fifteen scars from nine patients were treated with emulsified fat...". Though the two sentences are basically the same, the latter demonstrated our effort much better as it was started with fifteen not nine and our brain pays more attention to what we see first.

-If you have written a review article with many citations from a journal, submitting your paper to that journal will enhance the chance of acceptance. Editors like their journals to be cited, as this increases the impact factors of their journals. Also, if you are targeting a journal for publishing your work, having more references from that journal might increase the chance of acceptance by it.

-If your paper is rejected and you think the rejection is unfair, defend your paper by writing a letter to the editor and mention why you think the rejection is unfair. Sometimes, the editor reconsiders your paper for publication. You can include this statements in your letter: "As I believe that scientific arguments lead to the advancement of science, I would like to respond to the referees' criticisms as follows...". *J Am Acad Dermatol* is an example of a journal which frequently accepts logical appeals.

-Submitting a rejected paper to another journal without gaining the benefit from the comments and criticisms of the reviewers who have rejected the paper is definitely a foolish act.

-Submitting a rejected paper to another journal having a different style without changing your paper according to the instructions of the second journal makes the second editor think he is dealing with a paper considered unworthy for publication elsewhere and re-evaluating this paper may be a waste of time and energy.

-When you want to submit your rejected paper to another journal, if you have included the name of the first journal in the name of your paper file, rename your file and erase the name of the first journal. For example, if the file of your paper which is rejected by *Br J Dermatol* is named as "psoriasis BJD", delete BJD before submitting it to another journal, as the second editor may understand that it is a paper rejected by another journal and will look down on it.

-Usually it is easier to publish in recently launched journals than older ones.

-For getting information on the journals which have published papers from your country, search PubMed using PubMed Advanced Search Builder by limiting your search to papers having 'dermatology' and your country's name in their affiliations, e.g (Iran[Affiliation]) AND (dermatology[Affiliation]). This can be especially useful for authors from developing countries, as some journals may accept papers from these countries easier than other journals.

-If you cannot test your idea, you can publish it as a hypothesis. The journal *"Medical Hypotheses"* is dedicated to publishing this sort of papers. *FASEB* Journal also publishes hypotheses. You may also publish some of your hypothetical papers as Opinion, Commentary, or Letter to the Editor in other journals. However, I do not recommend writing many hypotheses; try to test your ideas instead. Also, keep in mind that many editors do not like publishing speculative papers; therefore, publishing hypotheses is not easy.

-In writing a hypothesis, it is important to magnify your supportive evidence by adverbs. For example, if nitric oxide is involved in the pathogenesis of alopecia areata and you would like to hypothesize a nitric oxide synthase inhibitor as a treatment for this condition, it is better to write "Nitric oxide is shown to be crucially involved in the pathogenesis of alopecia areata through the following mechanisms...".

-Try to choose a head-turning, captivating title for your paper. For example, if you are speculating for the first time that homocysteine can enhance skin ageing, it is better to choose "Homocysteine May Accelerate Skin Aging: A New Chapter in the Biology of Skin Senescence" as the title rather than "Homocysteine May Accelerate Skin Aging". Another example of a captivating title is: "Nicotinamide: A potential Addition to the Anti-Psoriatic Weaponry" rather than the ordinary title "Nicotinamide: A potential Addition to the Anti-Psoriatic Treatments".

-It is important to provide strong references for the notions you use for proposing a hypothesis. For example, in the nitric oxide synthase inhibitor hypothesis mentioned above, you should cite as many references as possible for the involvement of nitric oxide in the pathogenesis of alopecia areata, esp. citing the high-impact factor journals, to persuade the referees to accept your hypothesis. This is especially important if your hypothesis is strange and hard for the people to accept it.

-Check the title page of your paper meticulously for any error. Title page is like the window of a shop and any mistake in it can take a heavy toll on the fate of your paper.

-Publishing a negative result is very difficult, as editors enjoy publishing positive, moving results! If you have a negative result, you may still succeed in publishing it if you write your paper very well as a Letter (Research Letter or Letter to the Editor). In your cover letter to the editor, you should mention the importance of your negative result and even publishing negative results in general. For example, you can write that "Most editors would like to publish positive results. However, this causes a positive selection bias in the medical literature, which can have some dire consequences such as the waste of times, resources, and energies of the researchers who re-conduct the same research because of unawareness of the negative results already obtained by other researchers...". Moreover, you need to select an eye-catching title for your paper. For example, I chose this title for our paper reporting a negative result: "Clofazimine, an anti-mycobacterial with potent *in vitro* and *in vivo* leishmanicidal activity, is ineffective against cutaneous *Leishmania major* infection in humans" and published it in *J Am Acad Dermatol*. Another title, *e.g.* "Clofazimine is ineffective against cutaneous *Leishmania major* infections in humans" would be much less interesting. Moreover, it not only would not help in getting acceptance, but also may even be deterrent, as the reader may wrongly think it is evident that an anti-mycobacterial cannot work against a protozoal disease! As another pearl, very specific journals, esp. basic science journals interested in translational research, may be more welcoming towards negative results of clinical studies. For example, we succeeded to publish our negative result on serum magnesium concentrations in vitiligo patients in the journal *Magnesium Research* and another negative result on serum angiotensin converting enzyme levels in alopecia areata in *Enzyme Research*. Publishing these papers in clinical journals would have perhaps been very difficult, if not entirely impossible.

-Any rare case is not suitable for presentation as a case report. For example, if you see a case of progeria, one of the rarerst human diseases, you cannot present it as a case report because it is already mentioned in textbooks. However, if you notice an unreported sign in your progeria case, it will deserve publication.

-Some journals, such as *New England Journal of Medicine, Lancet, Dermatology Practical and Conceptual, Cutaneous Medicine and Surgery, JAMA Dermatology, etc.* accept interesting images with a description. You can publish your interesting clinical and pathologic images as a Clinicopathologic Challenge in some journals such as *International Journal of Dermatology, JAMA Dermatology, Dermatology Online Journal, etc.*

-I used to write my name in my papers as "Mohammad Reza Namazi", but I frequently noticed its incorrect PubMed-indexation as "M. Reza Namazi" and I had to email the indexers to correct it. Now, I prefer to write my name as "Mohammad R. Namazi" to avoid this problem.

-If you plan to get acceptance for competitive training courses, try to publish your papers in your own specialty field rather than the related disciplines. For example, I have published two papers in a high impact factor journal, *FASEB J*; however, if a professor in another country intends to evaluate my CV for a scholarship, being unaware of the importance of this journal, he will underevaluate me. Moreover, I believe that publishing a paper as a research letter in a high impact factor journal, like *J Am Acad Dermatol*, is better for a person's CV than publishing it as an original paper in a journal with a lower impact factor. The reason is that most professors are very busy, and they receive many applications. Therefore, they do not have enough time to evaluate your CV thoroughly. Usually, they do not scrutinize which paper is a research letter and which one is an original article. The names of the high impact factor journals are the factors which absorb their attention most.

-If you are co-authoring a paper with some people who you think may not observe the ethical codes and for the sake of gaining more credit may omit your name or give you a lower authorship rank, ask them about the status of the paper from time to time to send them the signal that the paper is important to you and you are serious about mentioning your name and your authorship rank on the paper.

- Writing a "Letter to the Editor" as a criticism of an already published paper will annoy the authors of the paper, even if they are very science-minded, and will negatively affect your relationship with them. Writing many critical "Letters" may negatively affect your CV, making the impression of a fussy or argumentative person.

-Including the name of a very famous person in your paper does not guarantee its publication in a targeted journal. There are some reasons for this, such as the blinded peer review system or the conflict between that person and the editor of the journal you are submitting the paper to.

-Once you receive the proof (galley proof), you may be allowed to add a short paragraph to your paper as "Note Added to the Proof", which will be printed at the end of your paper.

-Try to focus your research on just one subject or so, *e.g.* just on vitiligo. In this way, with time, you will be known as an expert on this subject. A big mistake of some researchers, esp. from the developing world, is that they research on multiple subjects. If you do so, you spend a lot of time and energy, but you end up becoming "the master of none"! Remember that laser is powerful because, in contrast to ordinary light, it is composed of just one wavelength not many and that the focused light coming from a magnifier has the power to burn while the ordinary light has not. Power comes from focusing!

- A useful tip for increasing your chance of getting acceptance for oral presentation and/or scholarship from a congress is that if your paper is accepted for publication in a prestigious journal, mention it at the end of your abstract.

-A few writing points:

Acknowledgment and Acknowledgement are both correct.

Table should be written with capital T, even in the middle of the text, *e.g.* The data are summarized in **T**able 1 (not table 1).

SUBJECT INDEX

A

Acid 15, 21, 22, 32, 41, 42, 43, 48, 51, 52, 54, 85, 87, 102, 106, 116, 129, 135, 138
  alpha hydroxy 43
  alpha-lipoic 32
  azelaic 52, 54, 106
  boric 85
  folic 116
  hyaluronic 129
  Pantothenic 15
  salicylic 21, 22, 41, 42, 43, 48, 51, 52, 54, 87, 102, 135, 138
  valproic 32
Acne 12, 47, 48, 49, 50, 54, 56, 59, 107
  inflammatory 59
  resistant 48, 107
Acne 16, 56
  prone skin 16
  vulgaris 56
Acquired immunity 91
ACTH stimulation test 28
Actinic keratosis 37, 137
Activation, fibroblast 130
Activity 5, 79, 92, 96, 101, 102, 136
  anti-tumor 92
  antioxidant 96
  matrix metalloproteinase 79
Acute 21, 28, 43
  electrolyte shifts 28
  exudative inflammation 21
  inflammatory stage 43
Adapalene cream 51, 52
Additive 44, 62, 133
  anti-pruritus effects 44
  keratolytic effects 62, 133
Adherence, therapeutic 90
Adiponectin 107
Agents 15, 27, 43, 44, 47, 50, 51, 54, 55, 60, 89, 94, 96, 99, 102, 106, 116, 121, 130
  anti-fungal 89

anti-inflammatory 43, 55, 130
  chemotherapy 116
  depigmenting 99
  immunosuppressive 27
  moisturising 60
Allergic rhinitis 45
Alopecia areata 29, 87, 88, 141, 142
  chronic 87, 88
  focal 29
  pathogenesis of 141, 142
Aluminium 135, 136
  chloride 136
  foil 135
Alzheimer's disease 93
Amitryptiline 32
Ammonium lactate 43
Amniotic membranes 36
Anagen 87
  follicles 87
  hair follicles 87
Anesthetic effect 19
Angiogenic properties 79
Angle closure glaucoma 46
Anterior uveitis 68
Anthralin 87
Anti-histamines 32, 45, 98
  ingested first-generation 45
  of choice for breastfeeding mothers 45
Anti-inflammatory effects 25, 26, 27, 51, 52, 54, 62, 130, 135
Anti-itch effect 19, 44
Anti-oxidant enzymes superoxide dismutase 102
Anti-platelet aggregation 127
Anti-psoriatic 142
  treatments 142
Antibodies 64
  anti-desmoglein 64
Anticholinergics 46, 65, 84
Antigen(s) 15, 38, 64, 91
  induced lymphocyte transformation inhibition 15

keratinocyte membrane 64
Apoptosis 99, 130
Atrophy, cause skin 29
Atropin in cold cream 136
Autoimmune disorder 101
Autoimmunity 113
Aven Cicalfate cream 135

B

Bandages, dry 123
Base, semiocclusive cream 62
Behcet's disease 68
Bitemporal thinning 111
Blocking testosterone 107
Botulinum toxin 130
Bradycardia 60
Breast cancer 108
Burning 16, 22, 32, 37, 72, 87, 125, 135
    dysesthesia 32
    sensation 16, 22, 125, 135

C

Callosities 15
Cancers, cervical 35, 36, 39
Carcinoma cuniculatum 36
Cardiac consultation 65
Carotid artery stenosis 118
Cholinergic 65
    agonists 65
    ocular 65
Chronic 70, 79, 125, 127, 135
    inflammatory condition 70
    lymphedema 135
    venous disorders 125, 127
    venous insufficiency 125, 127
    wounds 79
Cicamosa 130
Cinere intense hair repair 104
Clindamycine 136
Clobetasol cream 101
Clofazimine 85, 142
Clonidine 60, 136
Collagen fibers 56
Colonizing microflora 77
Combination 22, 32, 47, 51, 62, 74, 75, 85,
        108, 136, 137
    clindamycin-rifampin 137
    cyclosporine-methotrexate 74

Corona phlebectatica 125
Corticosteroids 21, 68, 130
    high-dose systemic 130
Cosmeceuticals 62
COVID-19 in-hospital mortality 91
Cryoglobulin 119
Cryotherapy 38, 41, 85, 135
Cutaneous ulcers 68
Cyclosporine 74, 75, 121, 134
    induced renal dysfunction 75
Cystoscopy 38

D

Damaged skin 14, 62
Dandruff complain 57
Daptomycine 136
Dehydration, reducing 48
Denaturing keratin 63
Dental floss 37
Depigmentation treatment 99
Depositions 93, 129
    excess collagen 129
Depression, respiratory 45
Dermal elastolysis 56
Dermatitis 16, 45, 75, 77, 89, 122, 123, 125,
        130, 136, 137
    acute 130
    atopic 16, 45, 75, 89
    lip licker 122
    seborrheic 77
Dermatomyositis 60
Dermatoses 22, 75
    acute 22
Dexpanthenol cream 14, 15, 62
Diabetes 60, 119, 127
Diabetic 79, 129
    foot ulcers 79
    nephropathy 129
Dilated vascular channels 75
Disease 7, 8, 28, 36, 45, 64, 65, 69, 70, 72, 74,
        75, 77, 83, 87, 101, 109, 111, 134, 138,
        140
    allergic 45
    autoimmune 87, 101
    cardiac 28, 83
    comorbid 72
    dry eye 109
    fatal blistering 64
    non-alcoholic fatty liver 109

oral 64
psychiatric 77
thyroid 111
transmitted 36
Disorders 32, 43, 46, 60, 119, 127
heart rhythm 32, 46
hyperkeratotic 43
immune 119
lymphatic 127
DNA damage 96
Downregulate hyaluronic acid expression 129
Drug(s) 12, 23, 32, 38, 84, 87, 111, 116, 119, 137
immunity-enhancing 38
nephrotoxic 119
resistant pathogens 137

E

Edema 125, 126, 127
peripheral 126
Effect 25, 26, 27, 28, 32, 43, 45, 46, 49, 57, 62, 91, 106, 127, 130
anti-acne 49
anti-androgenic 57, 106
anti-depressant 45
anti-inflammtory 130
anticancer 91
anticholinergic 32, 46
antihistamine 45
antimicrobial 62
cardiovascular 27
cytotoxic 91
glucocorticoid 25, 26, 28
keratolytic 43, 62
vasodilatory 127
Ehlers-Danlos syndrome 134
Elastic fiber degradation 56
Endothelial dysfunction 127
Epidermolysis bullosa 129, 130
Erectile dysfunction 127, 130
Erythema 60, 62, 68, 69, 101, 127, 135
elevatum diutinum 69
post-laser 135
solar 60
Erythroderma 27, 28
Erythrodermic psoriatis 75
Erythromycin 48, 49

F

Fibrosis, experimental pulmonary 129
Fibrotic processes 130
Fingertip dermatitis 122
Folliculitis 138
Functions, nerve-derived substances modulate sebocyte 57

G

Glaucoma 32
Glucocorticoid potencies 25
Glutathione peroxidase 102
Glycerin 14, 15, 18, 19, 41, 62, 63

H

Hair 104, 105, 111, 113, 129
bleached 104
damaged 105
disorders 111
line, frontal 113
proteins 105
transplantation 129
Hair loss 48, 106, 107, 108, 111
female pattern 108
severe androgenic 107
Hand dermatitis 137
Head lice infestation 81
Headache, severe acute 118
Heart failure 60, 118, 127
moderate congestive 60
renal failure/congestive 118
Hemolytic reaction 119
Hepatic 84, 116
disorder 84
function tests 84
toxicities 116
Hepatotoxicity 107
HIV, transmitting 36
Homocysteine 142
HPV 36, 38
infection 38
positive cases 38
vaccine 36
Human papilloma virus (HPV) 35, 36, 37, 38
Hydrogen peroxide 102
Hypercholesterolemia 46
Hyperhidrosis 136

facial 136
Hyperplasia 45
Hypertension 33, 65, 75, 119
  chronic 119
Hyperthyroidism 57
Hypertransaminasemia 107

I

IFN-gamma release assay 75
Infections 36, 38, 75, 89, 118, 137, 142
  chronic diabetic foot 137
  intestinal 36
  oral 36
  soft tissue 137
  viral 118
Inflammation 37, 77, 113, 122, 123, 124
  chronic 122
  lichenoid 113
  reducing 124
Inflammatory skin conditions 116
Inhibitor, nitric oxide synthase 141
Iron 112
  absorption 112
  deficiency 112
Irreversible joint damage 72
Ischemic ulcer 127
Itch 18, 19, 32, 46, 62, 71, 87, 93, 102, 130, 134
  resistant 134
  sensation 19
  severe 62
Itching 45, 125

K

Keratinocytes 15
Kidney failure, acute 119

L

Lesions 21, 38, 43, 68, 134
  nodular amyloidosis 43
  severe actinic purpuric 134
  thick hyperkeratotic 21
  urethral 38
  vascular 68
Lice 81
  head 81
  medicine 81

Lichen planopilaris 113, 114
Lipodermatosclerosis 125, 126
Liposomal amphotericin 85
Liver dysfunction 107

M

MBEH therapy 99
Mechanical tension 130
Medications 11, 12, 13, 21, 34, 37, 50, 62, 66, 71, 72, 74
  anti-psoriatic 74
Melanocytes 99, 100
Melanogenesis 102
Melasma, resistant 52
Mesotherapy 55
Mineralocorticoid effects 25, 28
Mometasone 22, 51, 52, 93, 94, 102
  cream 51, 52, 93, 94, 102
  ointment 22

N

Nail 71, 134
  psoriais, severe 134
  separation 71
Nausea 84, 116, 118
Nondermatologic conditions 27
Noreva Kerapil cream 43
Nutritional deficiencies 111

O

Ocular tolerance 61
Ointments, steroid 123
Oral 36, 64
  cancer 36
  candidiasis 64
  cavity 36
Osteoporosis 134

P

Pain 7, 32, 33, 42, 72, 84, 111, 118, 125, 127, 130
  abdominal 84
  acute 33
  joint 72
  neuropathic 32

Papules, follicular 56
Pathophysiology of psoriasis 140
Pelvic tumors 125
Petrochemical industry 16
Polymerase chain reaction (PCR) 38
Powder 22, 49, 51, 52, 89, 106
　clindamycin 49
　erythromycin 49
Pro-fibrotic factors 130
Pro-inflammatory cytokines 102, 129
Problem 28, 46, 84, 125
　cardiac 28
　cosmetic 125
　heart 84
　psychiatric 46
Psoriasis 70, 71, 72, 74, 75, 76, 123, 134, 137,
　140
　and pathomechanism 140
　and pathophysiology 140
　erythrodermic 123
　nail 71, 134
　symptoms 71
Psoriatic arthritis 72

R

Reactions 16, 21, 31, 60, 70, 84, 91, 118, 121
　allergic 16, 21, 121
　cell-mediated immune 91
　cutaneous drug 31
　photoallergic 60
Reactive oxygen species 96
Renal 24, 28, 34, 84
　damage 34
　disease 28
　failure 24, 84
Renin-angiotensin system inhibitors 119
Retinoid-associated irritation 94
Retinopathy 113
Rheumatoid arthritis 113
Risk 52, 126
　factors, cardiovascular 126
　thromboembolic 52

S

Scalp 72, 111
　inflammation 111
　psoriasis 72
Seborrhoeic dermatitis 77

Septicemia 74, 75, 119
Skin 14, 15, 47, 49, 50, 60, 61, 62, 71, 90,
　129, 135
　barrier function 15, 62
　dehydration 60
　dry 47, 49, 50
　dryness 14
　erythema 61
　inflammation 60
　irritate 71
　irritation 15, 90, 135
　scarring conditions 129
Skin diseases 1, 69, 77, 91
　inflammatory 77
　neutrophilic 69
Skin-lightening 52, 55
　agents 52, 55
　cream 55
Solar irradiation 101
Stress 3, 77, 89, 104, 111, 137
　emotional 137
　mechanical 104
　oxidative 111
Stroke risk factors 33
Symptoms, psychiatric 108

T

Tacrolimus cream 103
Tetracyclic anti-depressant 46
THAIS disease 133
Therapy 38, 46, 79, 80, 107, 119, 136
　hyperbaric oxygen 79, 80

U

Urokinase-type plasminogen activator 64

V

Vacuum-assisted closure (VAC) 79
Vascular 79, 125
　endothelial growth factor 79
　insufficiency 125

W

Water-resistant cream 61
Wounds 79, 89, 127, 129, 130
  fetal 129
  heal 130

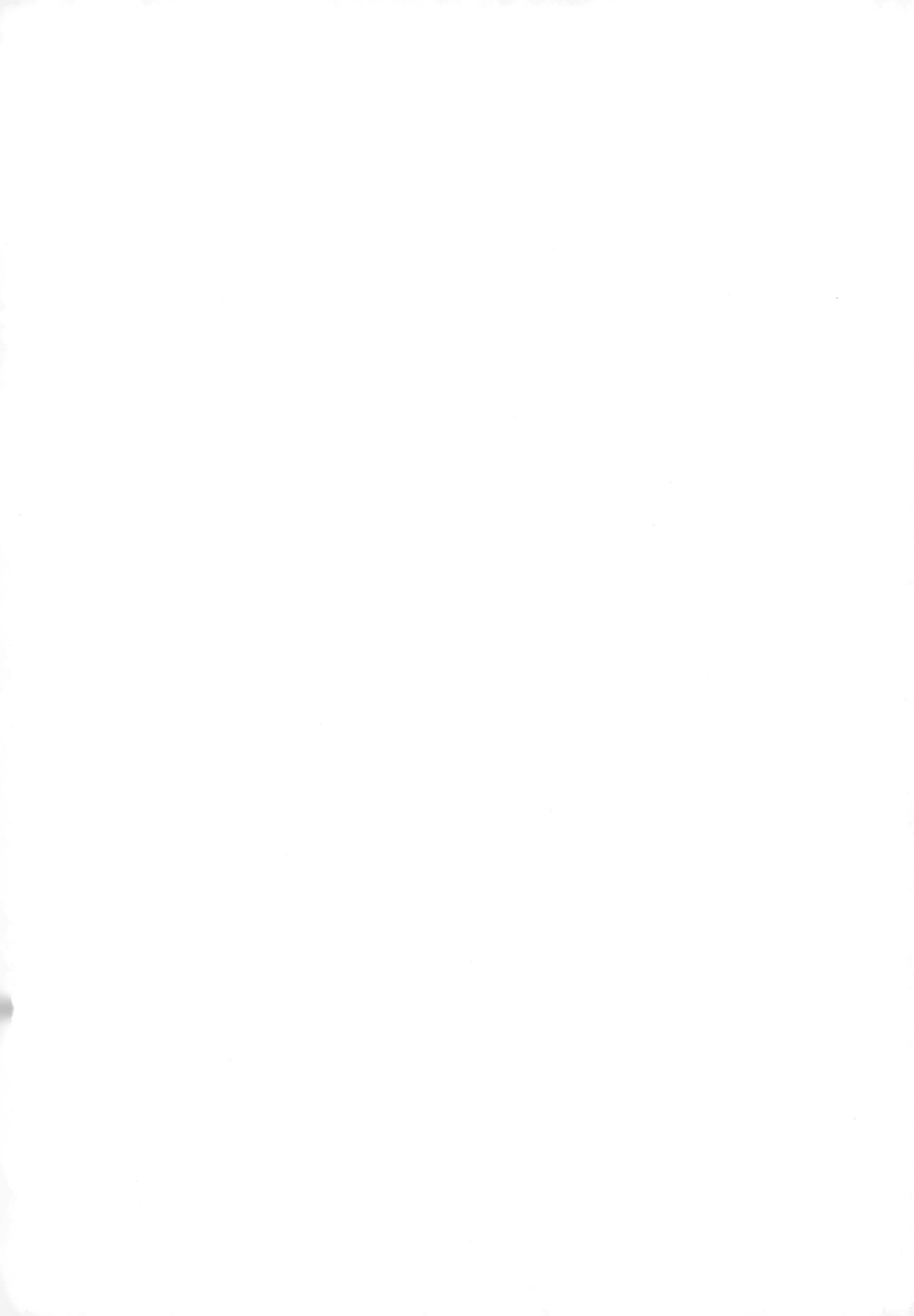

www.ingramcontent.com/pod-product-compliance
Lightning Source LLC
Chambersburg PA
CBHW041708210326
41598CB00007B/574